In order to help people with a mental illness, it is important to be able to understand and measure the severity of the experiences that they find distressing and disabling and which can affect their behaviour. SCAN is a set of instruments that provide a detailed and accurate picture of 'mental state'. The central method is an interview, the Present State Examination, which has been developed over 25 years; the current edition is the 10th. Patients find it appropriate and acceptable. A computerised form is available, which allows the organisation of algorithms that analyse the data and provide diagnoses according to the two internationally agreed systems, ICD-10 and DSM-IV. This reference manual describes the rationale and development of the SCAN system, its results, training methods and uses.

T0275855

Diagnosis and clinical measurement in psychiatry

Diagnosis and clinical measurement in psychiatry

A reference manual for SCAN

Edited by

J. K. Wing,

N. Sartorius

and

T. B. Üstün

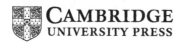
CAMBRIDGE
UNIVERSITY PRESS

CAMBRIDGE UNIVERSITY PRESS
Cambridge, New York, Melbourne, Madrid, Cape Town, Singapore, São Paulo

Cambridge University Press
The Edinburgh Building, Cambridge CB2 2RU, UK

Published in the United States of America by Cambridge University Press, New York

www.cambridge.org
Information on this title: www.cambridge.org/9780521434775

First published 1998
This digitally printed first paperback version (with corrections) 2006

A catalogue record for this publication is available from the British Library

Library of Congress Cataloguing in Publication data

Diagnosis and clinical measurement in psychiatry: a reference manual
for SCAN/PSE-10 / edited by J. K. Wing, N. Sartorius, and T. B. Üstün.
     p.   cm.
Includes index.
ISBN 0 521 43477 7 (hardback)
1. Mental status examination.   2. Psychodiagnostics.
3. Psychological tests.   I. Wing, J. K. (John Kenneth), 1923–   .
II. Sartorius, N.   III. Üstün, T. B.
[DNLM: 1. Mental disorders – classification.   2. Mental disorders – diagnosis.   3. Psychiatric status rating scales.   4. Psychological
tests.   5. Interview, psychiatric.   WM 15 D5355   1998]
RC386.6.M44D53   1997
616.89′075 – dc20
DNLM/DLC
for Library of Congress   96-26653 CIP

ISBN-13 978-0-521-43477-5 hardback
ISBN-10 0-521-43477-7 hardback

ISBN-13 978-0-521-03349-7 paperback
ISBN-10 0-521-03349-7 paperback

Contents

Authors and members of WHO SCAN Advisory Committee, 1996–1998

Professor P. Bebbington, Department of Psychiatry and Behavioural Sciences, Archway Wing, Whittington Hospital, Highgate Hill, London N19 5NF, UK.

Dr A. Bertelsen, Institute of Psychiatric Demography, Århus Psychiatric Hospital, DK-8240 Risskov, Denmark.

Professor J. L. Vázquez-Barquero, Hospital Universitario 'Marques de Valdeicilla', Faculdad le Medicina, 39000 Santander, Spain.

Dr. T. S. Brugha, Section of Social and Epidemiological Psychiatry, Department of Psychiatry, Leicester General Hospital, Leicester LE5 4PW, UK.

Dr. S. Chatterji, National Institute of Mental Health and Neurosciences, Department of Psychiatry, Post Bag No. 2979, Bangalore 560029, India.

Dr W. M. Compton III, Department of Psychiatry, Washington University School of Medicine, 4940 Children's Place, St Louis, Missouri 63110, USA.

Mr G. Der, MRC Medical Sociology Unit, University of Glasgow, Glasgow G12 8RZ, UK.

Dr Gyles Glover, Charing Cross and Westminster Medical School, London W6, UK.

Dr. A. Göğüs, Department of Psychiatry, Hacettepe University Medical School, 06100 Ankara, Turkey.

Professor G. L. Harrison, Professorial Unit, Mapperley Hospital, Porchester Road, Nottingham NG3 6AA, UK.

Dr V. Mavreas, Department of Psychiatry, University of Athens, Eginition Hospital, 74 Vas. Sophias Avenue, 11528 Athens, Greece.

Dr F. J. Nienhuis, Department of Social Psychiatry, PO BOX 30.001, 9700RB Groningen, The Netherlands. www.psy.med.rug.nl/0018

Professor C. Pull, Centre Hospitalier de Luxembourg, Service de Neuropsychiatrie, 4 rue Barblé, Luxembourg.

Dr A. Romanowski, The Johns Hopkins University, Department of

Psychiatry, Meyer Building, Room 4–181, 600 North Wolfe Street, Baltimore 21287, USA.

Professor N. Sartorius, Department of Psychiatry, University Hospitals, 16–18 Boulevard de St Georges, 1205, Geneva, Switzerland.

Dr A. Y. Tien, The Johns Hopkins University, School of Hygiene and Public Health Department of Mental Hygiene, 624 North Broadway, Baltimore, Maryland 21205, USA.

Professor J. K. Wing, College Research Unit, Royal College of Psychiatrists, 11 Grosvenor Cresent, London SW1X 7EE, UK.

Professor Y. Nakane, Nagasaki University School of Medicine, Department of Neuropsychiatry, 7–1, Sakamoto-machi, Nagasaki 852, Japan

World Health Organization

T. B. Üstün and J. Orley, Division of Mental Health and Prevention of Substance Abuse, WHO, Geneva 27, CH1211 Switzerland.

Up to date information concerning SCAN

Information concerning SCAN and its components – including the PSE-10 Interview Manual, Item Group Checklist, Clinical History Schedule, Glossary, Training Manual and software applications – is available on the WHO web site for SCAN with instructions on how to obtain them. If convenient, contact a SCAN Training and Reference Centre. A list of addresses is at page viii and is also included in the SCAN interview manual.

Alternatively, write to Doctor T. Bedirhan Üstün, Chief, Epidemiology, Classification and Assessment Unit, Division of Mental Health and Prevention of Substance Abuse, Room L3.19, WHO, CH-1211 Geneva 27, Switzerland.
Tel: +41.22.791.3609
Fax: +41.22.791.4885
E-mail: USTANT@WHO.CH

Preface

The reference manual for the ninth edition of the Present State Examination (PSE-9), together with an algorithm for deriving diagnoses according to the eighth edition of the International Classification of Diseases (ICD-8), was the first edition of the PSE to be published in full (1974). It was based on 15 or more years of development and experience, culminating in the use of the seventh and eighth editions in two large international research projects – the US–UK Diagnostic Project and the WHO International Pilot Study of Schizophrenia. Because PSE-9 is brief compared with its predecessors, and a 40-item version of it can be used by trained but non-clinical interviewers for screening purposes in two-stage population surveys, it has proved very popular. A voluminous scientific literature resulted and is still accumulating. However, the advent of consensus diagnostic algorithms, in DSM-III and its successors, and the provision of an international standard in ICD-10, meant that a compatible tenth edition of the PSE must be provided. This is now implemented as the main part of the SCAN.

The points made in the preface to the reference manual for PSE-9 remain relevant for SCAN/PSE-10. In particular, the principle of top-down application of diagnostic algorithms (at that time created from the prose descriptions in ICD-8; DSM-III was still 6 years away) to a database of ratings of clinical phenomena each differentially described in a Glossary, remains fundamental. Creating each database is a joint project between interviewer and respondent, and should be independent of preconceptions about classification. The independent diagnostic rules are then applied electronically. Both processes are being immensely simplified by the use of the computer-assisted PSE (CAPSE), the results from which can also be used to inform the respondent. CAPSE provides options for the analysis and presentation of symptomatic or diagnostic profiles based on one or a series of clinical interviews with one respondent, and also for analysis of data from groups of respondents. This ease of use and choice of outputs could not have been contemplated 23 years ago.

The final sentences of the original preface will serve to end this one also. 'The system can be improved by dropping some of the symptoms, adding others, polishing the definitions of others and, in general, coming closer to the truth. There will certainly be a need for a further edition eventually.'

J. K. Wing
College Research Unit
11 Grosvenor Crescent
London SW1X 7EE, UK

N. Sartorius
Department of Psychiatry
University Hospitals
16–18 Boulevard de St Georges
1205 Geneva, Switzerland

T. B. Üstün
Division of Mental Health and Prevention
of Substance Abuse,
World Health Organization,
Geneva 27, CH1211, Switzerland

Acknowledgements

The SCAN system has been developed in the framework of the World Health Organization (WHO) and National Institutes of Health (NIH) *Joint Project on Diagnosis and Classification of Mental Disorders, Alcohol and Drug Related Problems* (Principal Investigator, N. Sartorius, WHO). The development of SCAN was funded by WHO, NIH and Institutes employing collaborators who took part in the project.

SCAN had its origin in an existing instrument, the ninth revision of the Present State Examination (PSE). Its development is described in Chapter 2.

It is impossible to acknowledge the work of everyone who has participated during the past 16 years. No such enterprise can succeed without the advice, support and collaboration of many researchers, centres and agencies. Some, at least, are listed below.

Task force on diagnostic instruments:

J. K. Wing (Chair), M. von Cranach, C. Pull, L. Robins, H.-U. Wittchen, investigators from Field Trial Centres, staff of WHO and NIH

SCAN-1   1982–1992

WHO: N. Sartorius, A. Jablensky, T. B. Üstün, M. Grant
NIH: J. Blaine (NIDA), J. Burke (NIMH), B. Grant (NIAAA), R. Hirschfeld (NIMH), D. Regier (NIMH), L. Towle (NIAAA)

Field Trial Centres, principal investigators:

SCAN Field Trial Centres are listed on pages xv–xvi with centres that have been approved subsequently.

Contributions to the design and trial of particular parts of SCAN-1:

Alcohol and drug	T. Babor, A. Bertelsen, A. Göğüs, B. Grant, V. Nikolov, J. Strang, T. Tomov, J. L. Vázquez-Barquero
Cognitive symptoms	V. Mavreas, M. Roth, J. L. Vázquez-Barquero
Computer assisted interview	G. Glover
Computer design and programs	G. Der, N. Contracter, S. Gauthier, E. Glover
Consultants	H. Pfister, D. Rae
General editing	P. Bebbington, A. Bertelsen, T. Brugha, J. Cooper, J. Escobar, A. Farmer, V. Gentil, R. Giel, A. S. Henderson, A. Jablensky, T. B. Üstün
Glossary	T. Babor, P. Bebbington, R. Campbell, T. Üstün
Obsessional symptoms	G. Andrews
Print and graphic design	M. Locker, J. Stevenson, G. Der, J. Wing
Social impairment	L. Wing
Somatoform symptoms	P. Morosini, T. B. Üstün

General development of the SCAN-1 system and relevant training, co-ordination, data management and analysis: MRC Social Psychiatry Unit, Institute of Psychiatry, London.

Chief Editor: J. K. Wing.

SCAN-2.0   1992–1994

An editorial committee supervised changes necessary to incorporate the final revision of ICD-10 DCR: J. K. Wing (Chair), T. Babor, J. L. Vázquez-Barquero, P. Bebbington, A. Bertelsen, T. S. Brugha, S. Chatterji, W. M. Compton III, G. Harrison, V. Mavreas, A. Romanoski, N. Sartorius, A. Y. Tien and, at WHO, T. Üstün, A. Janca.

Textual changes were edited by A. Bertelsen, T. Brugha, S. Chatterji, W. M. Compton III, R. Y. Mehta, A. J. Romanoski and A. Y. Tien.

Development of computer programs for data entry, CAPSE, and ICD-10 and DSM diagnostic algorithms, was initiated by S. Chatterji,

G. Der, A. Y. Tien and T. B. Üstün. Inventa, Inc. of Bangalore, India (Principal programmers R. Ashok, C. P. Hari, and others) undertook the programming. S. Channabasavanna, R. Murthy and M. K. Isaac at the National Institute of Mental Health and Neurosciences in Bangalore provided support for editorial and programming work.

Administrative and secretarial assistance: R. Barrelet, J. Head (London), G. Covino, J. Wilson (Geneva), M. Brugha, I. Chenery (Leicester), D. Tien, M. Tseng (Baltimore).

SCAN-2.1   1994–1997

The WHO SCAN Advisory Committee supervised changes from SCAN version 2.0 to version 2.1: A. Bertelsen (Chair from July 1995), J. L. Vázquez-Barquero, T. S. Brugha, S. Chatterji, W. M. Compton III, F. J. Nienhuis, A. Göğüs, G. Harrison, V. Mavreas, A. Y. Tien, J. K. Wing and, at WHO, T. B. Üstün and J. Orley.

Errata lists were contributed by T. S. Brugha, J. L. Vázquez-Barquero, A. Bertelsen, C. G. Lyketsos, F. J. Nienhuis and A. Göğüs. Textual changes were edited by A. Bertelsen, T. S. Brugha, S. Chatterji and A. Y. Tien. The SCAN Advisory Committee (computer subcommittee) directed the further development of computer programs: A. Y. Tien (Chair), S. Chatterji, G. Der and T. Üstün. ICD-10 diagnostic algorithms were produced by S. Chatterji. DSM-IV algorithms were produced by S. Chatterji. DSM-IV algorithms were produced by G. Cai, W. Eaton, J. Lawler, A. Romanoski and A. Y. Tien. All algorithms were corrected by A. Bertelsen, T. S. Brugha, S. Chatterji, G. Der, W. M. Compton III, A. Romanoski and A. Y. Tien.

Administrative and secretarial help: D. Eggertsen (Århus), G. Covino, M. Brugha, I. Chenery (Leicester).

SCAN Training and reference centres (*field trial centres):

Details of the phone, fax, email and postal addresses and numbers of all SCAN centres are printed in the SCAN interview manual and Glossary, and can be updated on request to the Division of Mental Health and Prevention of Substance Abuse, WHO, Avenue Appia, Geneva, Switzerland.

Ankara, Turkey*	A. Göğüs
Århus, Denmark	A. Bertelsen
Athens, Greece*	V Mavreas

Baltimore, USA	A. Y. Tien
Bangalore, India*	M. K. Isaac
Beijing, China*	Shu Liang
Canberra, Australia*	B. Hughson
Cardiff, UK	A. Farmer
Farmington, USA*	J. Escobar, T. Babor
Geneva, Switzerland*	L. Barrelet
Groningen, Netherlands*	F. J. Nienhuis
Leicester, UK*	T. S. Brugha
London, UK*	P. E. Bebbington
Lübeck, Germany*	H. Freyberger
Luxembourg	C. Pull
Manchester, UK	L. Appleby
Mannheim, Germany*	K. Maurer
Nagasaki, Japan	Y. Nakane
Nottingham, UK*	G. Harrison
Perth, Australia	A. Jablensky
Santander, Spain*	J. L. Vázquez-Barquero
Sao Paolo, Brazil*	L. Andrade
Sofia, Bulgaria*	V. Nikolov
St Louis, USA	W. M. Compton
Verona, Italy*	M. Tansella

Chapter 9

Eric Glover (Biometrics, Institute of Psychiatry) made an important contribution to the ICD-10 programming, and Simon Shanks (Research Unit, Royal College of Psychiatrists) prepared the DSM-III-R program. We are also indebted to Robert Thomas (Advanced Systems Group, Warwick Research Institute) for designing the expert system.

Chapter 10

The need for revision of SCAN Version 1 was recognised by the WHO SCAN editorial committee in mid-1992. A small group consisting of T. S. Brugha (Leicester, UK), W. M. Compton (St Louis, USA) and A. Bertelsen (Århus, Denmark) was asked to take initial responsibility, with T. B. Üstün co-ordinating for WHO.

A preliminary draft was received and discussed by the SCAN

Editorial Group in February 1994, in London, and further modifications were introduced. SCAN version 2.0 was delivered to the publishers (APPI) in May 1994, and published and presented at the
meeting of the Association of European Psychiatrists in Copenhagen
in September that year. Some further changes and corrections were
agreed by the SCAN Advisory Committee meetings in Århus in July
1995, London in July 1996 and Luxemburg in November 1997, and
were incorporated as SCAN-2.1.

1 Measurement and classification in psychiatry

J. K. Wing, N. Sartorius and T. B. Üstün

Why measure and classify

The formulation and development of medical disease concepts requires an interaction between two essential components. One is reliable recognition and labelling of a cluster of physical and/or psychological characteristics, regarded as undesirable because of the distress or disability that accompanies them. Sometimes a single characteristic is enough. The other is the testing of hypotheses concerning the relationship of these characteristics to damage and dysfunction in underlying biological systems (pathology) and to their causes (aetiology).

The terminology of symptoms, syndromes and disorders implies a hierarchical link to biological causes which, even if currently unknown, will eventually be empirically demonstrated. This assumption has often proved unwarranted. Probably more such clusters have proved useless or misleading than have successfully survived the process of scientific testing.

The approach to the categorization of mental disorders adopted in the latest International Classification of Diseases (ICD-10; WHO, 1992) is therefore appropriately cautious. The term 'disorder':

is used to imply the existence of a clinically recognizable set of symptoms or behaviour that in most cases is associated with distress and with interference with functions, always at the individual level and often at the group or social level (but not the latter only).

To make an ICD-10 diagnosis of mental disorder is not, therefore, to specify the presence of a disease, but to recognise the presence of the designated syndrome. It does, however, allow hypotheses concerning a pathology or other biological abnormality to be tested. The epidemiology of the disorder can be investigated and may provide a basis for further hypotheses. Another obvious test of usefulness is whether making the diagnosis is helpful to the individual concerned. Does it accurately predict forms of treatment that reduce disability without harmful side-effects? Does it give some idea of the future course and outcome? Are there means of primary, secondary or tertiary prevention? These are matters for scientific inquiry.

At the very least, can the person afflicted and family carers be given the consolation that the condition has a name, that there are other people with similar problems and that experiences and methods of coping can be shared? The many charitable organisations that have been set up to help those who have a named syndrome, such as those attributed to Alzheimer, Asperger, Down, Kanner and Rett, demonstrate the value placed on the recognition of syndromes even at times when there was no hard-and-fast knowledge about causes and no cure was firmly available. The name is not a mere label, but an indispensable basis for communication and investigation.

A further benefit from testing disease theories is that there is often a bonus, both in the form of a reformulation of the original clinical syndrome and in the emergence of new knowledge of pathological, physiological, biochemical or etiological mechanisms that hitherto had been unsuspected. It is possible to hypothesise, on the basis of recently acquired biological knowledge, the existence of new syndromes within the old concepts.

Successful disease theories tend to evolve over time; from an initial association between a syndrome and a biological abnormality, towards a sophisticated complex of interlocking dimensional criteria based on deviations from normal biological functioning. The amount of knowledge involved in such concepts is immense by comparison with that in the initial categorical description. By the same token, the power to relieve suffering derived from the application of the knowledge may also increase dramatically (Häfner, 1987; Scadding, 1990).

This does not mean that it would have been possible to reach such a satisfactory formulation without having gone through a stage of simple categorisation, nor that disease categories can now be dismissed. To argue this would be to misunderstand the nature and value of scientific classification. Tycho Brahe and Linnaeus were part of a progressive scientific tradition, no less valuable because their contributions, if frozen into orthodoxy, would have persisted as a static and sterile preoccupation with description and classification. In fact, astronomy and botany could not have developed without them. Kepler and Darwin, and their successors in turn, would have had no foundations upon which to build.

The essentialist alternative to the empirical approach, in which disease entities are regarded as having an existence independent of the observer, was the main basis of medicine for 2000 years, notably in the Galenic humoral theory. But recent advances in knowledge have demonstrated the dimensional relationships underlying more and more apparently discrete clinical syndromes. Although we cannot avoid classifying, we can avoid reifying the resultant classes. Scientists should have no difficulty in passing from the categorical to the dimensional mode as it suits their purposes. Diabetes and hypertension are obvious examples.

International nosological systems, such as Chapter F of the new ICD-10, which provide standardised Diagnostic Criteria for Research (DCR; WHO, 1993) to guide clinical recognition of the syndromes of mental disorder, serve essential public-health and scientific purposes. It is necessary to use them sensibly and work to improve them. But they can only help to further knowledge if two conditions are met. First, and more important, the rules must be applied to a base of clinical observations ('symptoms and signs') that accurately reflect the condition of the patient. In other words, the application of standard rules does not of itself guarantee accuracy. Second, the resulting categories should not be regarded as disease entities, but as technical aids for testing clinical hunches and research hypotheses, and for providing good-quality records that can be used for public-health and epidemiological purposes.

This book describes the development and use of methods that help to ensure the fulfilment of both these essential conditions: the reliable and accurate description of symptoms and syndromes, and the testing of hypotheses concerning their relationship to damage and dysfunction in underlying biological systems.

It should be added that this approach does not in any way suggest that environmental influences are irrelevant, or deny their common role in causing, exacerbating or otherwise influencing the expression of symptoms, syndromes and disorders.

The development of psychiatric syndromes

The syndromes of 'schizophrenia', as described by Emil Kraepelin (1896) and Eugen Bleuler (1911), and the syndromes of 'autism', as described by Leo Kanner (1943) and Hans Asperger (1944), illustrate the fitful progress made in the clinical description of two groups of severely disabling mental disorders.

The importance of labels: early childhood autism

The problems of defining and labelling syndromes are clearly illustrated in the case of 'early childhood autism'. Victor, the 'wild boy of Aveyron' first described with stunning clarity by J. M. G. Itard in his reports of 1801 and 1806 (Lane, 1977), provides an illustration. The phenomena delineated by Itard are as recognisable now as they were then, but, because he did not formulate the abnormal behaviours as symptoms, nor name them as a syndrome, it was not recognised that the techniques he used could be generalised to a class of children who were not simply mentally retarded in a global fashion but had highly specific impairments. It was not until Kanner described the phenomena and pointed out the similarities between them (only eleven children, but that was enough), and Asperger described in equally convincing manner a variant of the same set of problems in young men (Frith, 1991; Wing, 1981, 1996), that the syndrome and its boundaries could be investigated epidemiologically, and its relationship to diseases of known etiology and to intellectual disability more generally could be elucidated.

The development of the concept also illustrates the dangers that can follow the adoption of a name. Kanner used Bleuler's term 'autism' to label the syndrome. The confusion with 'childhood schizophrenia' still persists, but both DSM-III-R and ICD-10 now distinguish between the two types of syndrome. Autism and schizophrenia may yet prove to be linked (Frith and Frith, 1991; Frith, 1992) but the principle involved in separating them for classification purposes is important. It is simpler to link categories at a higher level than to distinguish between them once they are merged. It must remain possible to retrieve and study the elements right down to symptom level.

The importance of labels: schizophrenia

Schizophrenia is a condition at present defined only in terms of certain abnormalities of experience and behaviour. With only conjectural underpinning in biological knowledge, there is room for a wide range of opinion as to which elements should be included or excluded. Two decades before Emil Kraepelin's views became influential, there was much the same discussion as now concerning the value of classifying severe mental disorders. The adherents of one school argued for the concept of a unitary psychosis; pointing out that there is an infinite variety of experience and behaviour and that to delineate boundaries between named classes is as fruitless as to try to classify the shapes of clouds. States of madness dissolved into each other, with or without a temporal sequence. Some proponents held that all mental illness began as melancholia and progressed through paranoia to dementia; others that virtually any sequence could occur.

Clouds can usefully be classified. The clarification in the fifth and sixth (1899) editions of Kraepelin's textbook brought to an end a period of chaos and introduced a simple, though crude, distinction between conditions characterised by mental deterioration, such as catatonia, hebephrenia and dementia phantastica, and the more periodic forms of mania and melancholia. He also hypothesised different causes for the two new 'disease entities'. The formulation was thankfully adopted because of its convenience.

The form in which dementia praecox has remained a dominant feature of psychiatric nosology is, of course, Eugen Bleuler's creation. The convenience of the new name, 'schizophrenia', must have played a large part in its acceptance, as did the fact that the connotations of the term 'dementia' seemed to have been dropped. Nevertheless, Bleuler's primary symptom was cognitive – loosening of the associations. This was his link to the biological origins of schizophrenia and also, through 'psychic complexes', to the disorders of affectivity, ambivalence, autism, attention and will. Catatonia, delusions, hallucinations and behavioural disturbance he regarded as accessory. These theoretical assumptions held for the largest sub-group, latent schizophrenia.

Bleuler's concept was subsequently used in markedly different ways. Under the influence of psychoanalysis in the United States, the least differentiated forms – latent and simple schizophrenia – dominated diagnosis to such an extent that descriptive psychopathology was derided and neglected. A similarly broad and vague approach to diagnosis in the Soviet Union, notably under the influence of the Moscow school, this time with a supposedly biological basis, was exploited for political purposes.

At a symposium held on the occasion of the 600th anniversary of the University of Heidelberg, a later occupant of Kraepelin's Chair, Werner Janzarik, described the history and discussed the problems of the concept of schizophrenia. He began his paper with the incontrovertible observation that the history of schizophrenia is the history of the clinical syndromes that were 'only gradually, and at a relatively late period, grouped under the new designation after numerous differentiations and reclassifications.' He ended the lecture with the statement: 'So far, there is no conclusively defined disease known as schizophrenia. The history of the concept is a history, not of medical discoveries, but of the intellectual models on which the orientation of psychiatry is based' (Janzarik, 1987).

The US–UK Diagnostic Project (Cooper et al., 1972) and the International Pilot Study of Schizophrenia (IPSS: WHO, 1973), in which the seventh and eighth editions of the Present State Examination (PSE: Wing, Cooper and Sartorius, 1974) were used, were set up as part of the reaction against the use of terms like 'schizophrenia' without any technical provenance. The studies demonstrated the extent to which such a diagnosis in the USA and USSR was broader and less definable compared with usage elsewhere. The strong resurgence of public-health psychiatry in the USA and the growth of biological psychiatry led to the creation of DSM-III and its subsequent editions, DSM-III-R (APA, 1987) and DSM-IV (APA, 1994), which provided top-down algorithms for classification that set real technical standards. ICD-10 (1993) moved in the same direction by providing international standards for Chapter F (WHO, 1993).

The limitations of these rule-based nosologies are obvious and accepted. A paper on possible future criteria for schizophrenia (Flaum and Andreasen, 1991) illustrates the problem. DSM-III-R, ICD-10 and three proposed options for DSM-IV were compared. It is clearly unlikely that one of these five sets of rules will be found to represent the clinical manifestations of a disease process, while the other four are not. 'State-of-the-art' rules formulated in the absence of external validating criteria are likely to be fragile and transitory unless there is a consensus among professional opinion that they should only be used in order to exploit the advantages for clinical comparability, professional education and scientific study provided by a reference classification.

Within these limits, the ICD-10 rules should remain the world standard until the next revision, to be used irrespective of whatever local or hypothesis-based criteria are used in addition. However, there remains the necessity to define and measure the phenomena on which the rules should operate.

International Classification of Diseases, tenth edition, ICD-10

The term 'disorder', as used in ICD-10, is a higher order equivalent to 'syndrome'. The structure of Chapter F does not conform to Hempel's ideal classification (1959), which is 'mutually exclusive and jointly exhaustive'. Such a structure is based on unattainable Aristotelian verities. Chapter F is one of 21 chapters in ICD-10, each using several axes of classification; some based on aetiology, some on pathology, some on syndrome. ICD-10 represents a stage in a gradual evolution that will continue as long as distressing and disabling disorders persist. The top-down classifying criteria for Chapter F make diagnoses more internationally comparable, thus enhancing clinical, educational, public health and research functions. That is good progress. But it is essential that the rules are applied to a base of clinical observation that accurately reflects the condition of the patient.

Categories and dimensions

As disease theories become more successful in providing a solid basis of knowledge about abnormalities of biological and psychological functioning, the dimensional aspects of measurement within and between clinical syndromes become apparent. Both modes of measurement are necessary for advance, and it should be possible to move from one to the other as appropriate, without any sense of incongruity. This is as true of mental disorders as it is of a condition like diabetes. A system of clinical measurement cannot be purely categorical or purely dimensional (Wing, 1995). The most obvious example of the dimensional approach is in defining severity of symptom types, whether for investigation, for treatment purposes or for the assessment of outcomes. But the symptoms themselves must first be defined.

Defining symptoms

The formulation and development of medical disease concepts requires an interaction between reliable recognition and labelling of one or a cluster of physical and/or psychological characteristics (regarded as undesirable because of the distress or disability that accompanies them) and demonstrable damage and dysfunction in underlying biological systems (pathology and/or aetiology). Medical terminology tends to label many such characteristics as 'symptoms' if a hypothetical link has been suggested, even when the evidence for it is inconclusive. The usage is so universal that it is adopted here. However, the caveat stated at the beginning of this chapter, that many such hypotheses have proved false, and even harmful when acted upon, must be kept in mind.

Undesired or undesirable physical symptoms are easier to define and recognise than psychological or behavioural equivalents, but a physical characteristic (sweating for example) is not necessarily symptomatic of a disorder simply because it *is* clearly 'physical'.

On the other hand, the closer the definitions of an abnormal subjective experience comes to what Lewis (1953) called a 'psychological dysfunction', because it is defined in terms of deviation from a standard of normal psychological functioning, the more easy it is likely to be to find a link to an abnormality of biological function. For example, a description of thoughts or impulses intruding into the mind against conscious resistence has long been familiar to psychiatrists who make a practice of listening in detail to the unpleasant experiences described by their clients. The name 'obsession' is a convenient label, which can be given a precise definition that differentiates it from other symptoms such as phobia or thought insertion (see Chapter 4). Thought insertion can similarly be differentially defined, and there are already testable theories of how it might be linked through a neuropsychological intermediary to neural processes (Frith and Frith, 1991; Frith, 1992).

The obverse is also true. Symptoms should be defined as far as possible without recourse to purely social factors in the definition. Shoplifting and vandalism, for example, are undesirable behaviours, defined in purely social terms, and relatively easy to define reliably. Biological theories can be invoked to help explain some aspects in some people, but are not likely to account for a useful proportion of the variance. The more exclusive the social component in defining deviance, the less applicable is a symptom label.

The problems of defining individual symptoms (and problem behaviours, often called 'signs') are considered in Chapter 4, which describes the SCAN Glossary.

Clusters or syndromes

Some symptoms are clearly members of a group because they have a core quality in common but manifest it in different ways. Obsessional symptoms, for example, have as a core quality the characteristic of intrusion into consciousness against the person's active willed resistance. But the content of the obsession varies widely. Many types of delusion, hallucination, phobia etc, are like this.

Another characteristic that helps, if present, to give solidity to a syndrome construct is when individual symptoms that are not apparently members of the same group nevertheless tend to occur together. The negative and positive symptoms 'of schizophrenia', for example, are so called because they do tend to coexist, and are thus thought likely to be related in some basic way.

Symptoms may also tend to occur in sequence rather than (or as well as) together, i.e. as a syndrome over time. There may be a recognisable 'natural' syndromatic course, episodic or developing, and also perhaps a characteristic outcome. Such syndromes have been refined over a century and a half of clinical observation, and elegantly described in such classics as Jaspers' General Psychopathology. On the whole, they have been supported by statistical analyses.

The social context of diagnosis

Diagnosis and treatment are central, though by no means exclusively, to the medical role. That is why, ostensibly at any rate, patients consult doctors. But these functions provide the occasion for others. Doctors should be familiar with the range of human experience and behaviour. Many of them should be able to take on something of the role of counsellor, befriender, teacher, psychotherapist, social worker or advocate. Moreover, diagnosis is at least as much to do with ruling out disease explanations as with establishing that one or other of them would prove useful for helping a patient.

The problems brought to psychiatrists are therefore far from exclusively biological. Biological abnormalities can have social causes; many biological systems depend for their proper functioning on interaction with the psychosocial as well as the physical environment; and social influences can amplify biological impairments. The extent to which an individual is socially disabled depends, in addition, on psychosocial factors such as disadvantage and public, family and self attitudes. The resulting problems of classification and measurement of long-term psychiatric disorders have been discussed elsewhere (Wing, 1992, 1995,; WHO, 1980).

Scientists must nevertheless try to keep the various factors contributing to social disablement theoretically separate, since they are likely to have different causes and practical effects and to require different types of intervention. This conclusion can be applied to most psychiatric syndromes, from phobias to dementia. The more clearly symptoms are described, and the more precisely the rules for grouping them into syndromes are specified, the more comparable will be tests of hypotheses of all kinds.

References

American Psychiatric Association (1987) *Diagnostic and statistical manual of mental disorders*, third edition – revised. Washington, DC: APA.

American Psychiatric Association (1994) *Diagnostic and statistical manual of mental disorders*, fourth edition. Washington, DC: APA.

Asperger H. (1944) Die autistischen Psychopathen im Kindesalter, *Archiv für Psychiatrie und Nervenkrankheiten*, 117: 76–136.

Bleuler E. (1911) Dementia praecox oder die Gruppe der Schizophrenien. In: Aschaffenburg G. (Hgr) *Handbuch der Psychiatrie*, Specieller Teil, 4. Abt. 1.Halfte. Leipzig: Deuticke.

Cooper J. E., Kendell R. E. Gurland B. J., Sharpe L., Copeland J. R. M. and Simon R. (1972) Psychiatric diagnosis in New York and London. London: Oxford University Press.

Flaum M. and Andreason N. C. (1991) Diagnostic criteria for schizophrenia and related disorders. *Schizophrenia Bulletin*, 17: 133–56.

Frith C. (1992) *The cognitive neuropsychology of schizophrenia*. Hove: Erlbaum.

Frith C. D. and Frith U. (1991) Elective affinities in schizophrenia and childhood autism. In: Bebbington P. (ed.) *Social psychiatry. Theory, methodology and practice*, pp. 65–88. New Brunswick and London: Transaction Publishers.

Frith U. (ed.) (1991) *Autism and Asperger syndrome*, Cambridge University Press.

Häfner H. (1987) The concept of a disease in psychiatry. *Psychological Medicine* 17: 11–14.

Hempel C. G. (1959) Introduction to problems of taxonomy. In: Zubin J.

(ed.) *Field studies in the mental disorders.* New York: Grune and Stratton.

Itard J. M. G. (1801, 1807) Memoire et rapport sur Victor de l'Aveyron. In: Maison L. (ed.) *Les enfants sauvages.* 1964. Paris: Union Generale d'Editions.

Janzarick W. (1987) The concept of schizophrenia. History and problems. In: Häfner H., Gattaz W. F. and Janzarik W. (eds.) *Search for the causes of schizophrenia*, pp. 11–18. Heidelberg: Springer-Verlag.

Jaspers K. (1946) *Allgemeine Psychopathologie.* Heidelberg: Springer-Verlag.

Kanner L. (1943) Autistic disturbances of affective contact. *Nervous Child*, 2: 217–50.

Kraepelin E. (1896) *Psychiatrie*, 5te Auflage, pp. 426–41. Leipzig: Barth.

Lane H. (1977) *The wild boy of Aveyron.* London: Allen and Unwin.

Lewis A. J. (1953) Health as a social concept. *British Journal of Sociology*, 4: 109–24.

Scadding J. K. (1990) The semantic problems of psychiatry. *Psychological Medicine*, 20: 243–48.

Wing J. K. (1976) Kanner's syndrome. A historical introduction. In: Wing L. (ed.) Early childhood autism, pp. 3–14. Oxford: Pergamon.

Wing J. K. (1992) Social consequences of severe and persistent psychiatric disorders. In: Leff J. and Bhugra D. (eds.) *Principles of social psychiatry.* London: Blackwell.

Wing J. K. (1995) Concepts of schizophrenia. In: Hirsch S. R. and Weinberger D. (eds.) *Schizophrenia*, chapter 1. Oxford: Blackwell.

Wing J. K., Cooper J. E. and Sartorius N. (1974) *The description classification of psychiatric symptoms. An instruction manual for the PSE and CATEGO system.* London: Cambridge University Press.

Wing L. (1981) Asperger's syndrome. *Psychological Medicine*, 11: 115–29.

Wing L. (1996) *The Autistic Spectrum.* London: Constable.

World Health Organization (1973) *The international pilot study of schizophrenia.* Geneva: WHO.

World Health Organization (1980) *International classification of impairments, disabilities and handicaps.* Geneva: WHO.

World Health Organization (1990) *International classification of diseases*, tenth edition. Geneva: WHO.

World Health Organization (1993) *International classification of diseases*, tenth edition. Chapter F. Mental and behavioural disorders. Diagnostic Criteria for Research. Geneva: WHO.

2   The PSE tradition and its continuation in SCAN

J. K. Wing

Introduction

It was suggested in Chapter 1 that disease concepts evolve over time. When mature (which is not to say immutable), they are states of somatic and psychological dysfunction attributable to a known pathogenesis, with a known pattern of recognition, course and outcome in the absence of modifying factors. The effects of the physical, social and psychological environment in causation, treatment and care are also known. Few disease concepts have reached the end of this evolution. Most psychiatric complaints are still in the early stages, so much so that ICD terminology refers to them only as 'disorders'. To make a 'psychiatric diagnosis', therefore, is to hypothesise, on the basis of incomplete information (as a minimum an observable pattern of symptoms and signs), that further knowledge will become available through the usual pattern of scientific research and clinical observation.

The more clearly symptoms are described, and the more precisely the rules for grouping them into syndromes are specified, the more comparable will be tests of hypotheses of all kinds. Validity, in terms of a demonstrable and replicable relationship to some independent criterion, can sometimes be demonstrated even when the manifestations are diverse and variable, but it would not be sensible to rely only on that chance. This is why it is necessary, not only to use the set of classifying rules in ICD-10, but also to provide for international use a set of differential definitions for each of the symptoms specified and for many that are not specified. It will be possible to apply other sets of rules as well, and to compare the results of hypothesis testing. Scientific examination of diagnostic concepts will then be possible in psychiatry as in other branches of medicine.

The history of the PSE

The development of a set of instruments intended to serve these purposes was made necessary by the research that had been undertaken in the Social Psychiatry Research Unit of the UK Medical Research Council 10 years following its foundation in 1948 (O'Connor, 1968). Several scales were available that quantified the behaviour and, to a lesser extent, the symptomatology of patients (Lorr, 1966; Venables, 1957; Venables and O'Connor, 1959; Wittenborn, 1955). The resulting scores were often analysed statistically in order to produce clinical groupings; for example, 'perceptual distortion'. The results were relatively reliable and precise compared with clinical procedures (Foulds, 1965; Kreitman, 1961) but the categories did not look very different from clinical syndromes already in use.

A simple descriptive categorisation of chronic schizophrenia was constructed, based on four symptoms commonly seen in mental hospital patients in those days, and rated at a semi-standardised interview. The items were flatness of affect, poverty of speech, incoherence of speech, and coherently described delusions and hallucinations (Venables and Wing, 1962; Wing, 1959, 1961, 1962).

The procedure was then extended to cover psychotic symptoms in greater detail, and sections dealing with neurotic symptoms were added to produce a further schedule which was later designated the third edition of the Present State Examination or PSE. This was rapidly expanded and reorganised during intensive studies between 1963 and 1966, and the results of wide-ranging tests of the third to fifth editions, based on interviews with 172 people in ambulatory, day and ward settings, were published (Wing et al., 1967). Reliability on scores was high, apart from the score on anxiety. Agreement on clinical diagnoses made independently of each other by the five psychiatrists taking part (all trained in the same school) was also high, although no standardised definitions of the symptoms or specification of the classifying rules, was attempted.

PSE-7 and 8. The US–UK and IPSS studies

An expanded sixth edition of the PSE was rapidly modified for use in two large international studies – the US–UK Diagnostic Study (Cooper et al., 1972) and the International Pilot Study of Schizophrenia (WHO, 1973, 1979). Reliability was satisfactory in both projects and others conducted elsewhere (Kendell et al., 1968; Luria and Berry, 1979; Luria and McHugh, 1974; Wing, Cooper and Sartorius, 1974). Both projects concentrated on the differential diagnosis of schizophrenia, particularly from affective disorders.

The central result of the US–UK study, using PSE-7 and PSE-8, was that the team of research psychiatrists, examining patients on both sides of the Atlantic, diagnosed far fewer schizophrenic disorders than their hospital counterparts in the USA, while agreeing more closely with hospital clinicians in the UK. The PSE profiles confirmed that New York hospital diagnoses of schizophrenia were substantially broader. This has no implications for validity in the strict sense, but does indicate that the boundaries of the disorder were, at that time, drawn so differently that the results of studies into causes, treatments and outcomes might well not be comparable if based on hospital diagnoses in New York and London.

The version developed for use in the IPSS (PSE-8) was extensively tested, discussed, translated and back-translated, and was found acceptable by patients and doctors. The IPSS investigators were a much larger and more diverse group than those of the US–UK study. They came from psychiatric departments in Århus, Agra, Cali, Ibadan, London, Moscow, Prague, Taipei and Washington. The result, however, was very similar. Centres in Moscow and Washington used a much broader definition of schizophrenia than the other seven, when PSE profiles were studied.

PSE-9

From the point of view of improving the PSE, three major lessons were learned from the IPSS:

(i)   a glossary of differential definitions should be provided as a basis for training courses;

(ii)   additional schedules would be needed to allow the rating of previous episodes of disorder and possible causes and pathologies;

(iii)   algorithms for classifying from PSE item profiles into ICD-8 diagnostic categories should be provided, in order to give a standard of reference in addition to (not as a substitute for) clinical diagnosis.

These features were incorporated into PSE-9, which was short, only 140 items derived from the 500 items of its predecessor. Each was given a differential definition in the Glossary. Together with a Syndrome Check List for previous episodes, an Aetiology Schedule and the CATEGO-4 computer program, the new system filled most of the gaps in the old (Wing, Cooper and Sartorius, 1974). The output included a profile of precursors to diagnosis, as well as a single tentative category and a choice of scoring systems.

A further innovation was the Index of Definition (ID), which provided a means of differentiating eight levels of confidence that sufficient symptoms were present to allow a diagnosis of one of the 'functional' categories of ICD-8 (Wing, 1976; Wing et al., 1978). The ID has subsequently been used, with some success, also as a measure of general severity. It is highly correlated with total score, due mainly to the fact that the upper levels (though not based on scores) do represent a hierarchy of disorders in terms of severity.

Three other modifications were found useful: a brief form, using only 10 items to identify 'cases' with remarkable success (Cooper and MacKenzie, 1981); a technique for ascertaining lifetime prevalence (McGuffin, Katz and Aldrich, 1986); and a change rating scale, using PSE-9 items, for monitoring clinical progress over time (Tress et al., 1987).

Publishing the PSE for the first time, after 10 years of development, provided an opportunity to state the aims of the system, summarise its limitations and advantages and specify the relationship between the PSE text and Glossary (Wing, 1983). These have not changed since, and are specified below for the successor system. Reliability remained high (Cooper et al., 1977; Lesage et al., 1991; Rogers and Mann, 1986; Wing et al., 1977).

The system has been used in numerous studies in most corners of the world, both in sample population surveys and in experimental research (e.g.: Bebbington et al., 1981; Dean et al., 1983; Henderson et al., 1979; Huxley et al., 1989; Knights et al., 1980; Lehtinen et al., 1990; Okasha and Ashour, 1981; Orley and Wing, 1979; Sturt, 1981; Urwin and Gibbons, 1979).

One unexpected limitation has been appreciated after hard experience, and should be borne in mind for the future. There has been a tendency to regard the CATEGO-4 output as equivalent to a diagnostic entity rather than as a rich and varied psychometric profile. That was far from the authors' intention (Wing, 1983). A central principle was that the system could not 'make a diagnosis' in that sense. The people who use it are responsible for interpreting the results according to their judgement of the adequacy of the interview, the quality of the data recorded and the choice of outputs from the computer analysis. Most of the output consists of profiles of scores or prefinal categories, with only one 'final' category that can be interpreted as a diagnosis if the user so decides.

Rose (1992) has made the point that diagnosis 'splits the world into two'; those who have, and those who do not have, a disorder. But most problems have continuous distributions. The PSE was not originally designed as a diagnostic instrument, but, in the course of its development as a comprehensive clinical tool, it came to provide a database capable (in addition to its psychometric properties) of expanding to exploit the more exacting algorithms presented in DSM-III.

PSE-10 and SCAN

More than 15 years of experience with the PSE-9 system provided a mass of suggestions for improvement. Preparations for a tenth edition were started in 1980 in anticipation of ICD-10 (Jablensky et al., 1983). The major emphasis of correspondents was on broadening the content, both by returning to the larger item-pool of PSE-7 and PSE-8, and by adding new sections to cover somatoform, dissociative and eating disorders, alcohol and drug misuse, and cognitive impairments. However, the PSE-9 principles continued to guide the new developments.

A second suggestion was that an extra rating point was needed to extend the 0–1–2 scales of severity used for most PSE-9 items, allowing a mild or 'sub-clinical' level to be used, particularly in population surveys.

A third, very obvious, requirement, was for a better technique for rating previous episodes of disorder, adding other items relevant to the history and to etiology, and processing all the resulting information by means of one set of computer programs.

The widespread acceptance and use of DSM-III-R meant that the database must contain all the clinical and course criteria specified in its manual, as well as those being developed for ICD-10, and that the new CATEGO-5 algorithm must contain both sets of classifying rules.

Finally, however, users made it clear that they would wish relevant items in PSE-10 to be convertible into PSE-9 equivalents, so that the CATEGO-4 program could be applied to produce output comparable with data from earlier studies.

The development of SCAN

The framework for the development of SCAN was the Joint Project on Diagnosis and Classification of Mental Disorders, Alcohol- and

Drug-Related Problems (Principal Investigator, N. Sartorius, WHO). This was a partnership between WHO and the US Alcohol, Drug Abuse and Mental Health Administration (ADAMHA) and was funded by these organizations, the UK Medical Research Council (MRC) and Institutes employing collaborators in the work. A Task Force on Diagnostic Instruments was set up in 1980 to develop further two instruments already in wide international use. The first was the Diagnostic Interview Schedule (DIS), which eventually became the Composite International Diagnostic Interview (CIDI, 1995). The second was PSE-9, which became the Schedules for Clinical Assessment in Neuropsychiatry (SCAN). A third instrument, the International Personality Disorder Examination (IPDE, 1992), was subsequently added.

A pilot version of PSE-10 was devised and used in a study of the need for care and services of long-term attenders at day hospitals and day centres in Camberwell, a deprived area of south-east London (Brugha et al., 1988). Some interesting results from this precursor are presented in Chapter 8. The experience, together with suggestions and comments from international reviewers whose opinions were canvassed by the WHO/ADAMHA Task Force, led to further additions and modifications (Wing et al., 1990). The resulting instrument (SCAN version 0, or SCAN-0, with CATEGO-5, February 1988) was used in international field trials to test reliability between interviewer and observer and between two interviewers over time, and general practicality in use across a wide range of disorders. Subsequent changes in the sections dealing with the use of alcohol and other drugs, eating and obsessional disorders, and cognitive impairments, led to further trials. The results of these tests are presented in Chapter 8.

SCAN was redesigned in the light of these experiences. In 1992, version 1 (SCAN-1), with its computer-assisted form CAPSE-1 (see Chapter 9), was different in many ways from SCAN-0 used in the 1988 trials. However, no sooner had these changes been assimilated and late changes to the Diagnostic Research Criteria of ICD-10 been incorporated, than DSM-IV began to emerge over the horizon. It was not until September 1994 that SCAN-2.0 (see Chapter 10) was presented at a meeting of the Association of European Psychiatrists in Copenhagen. With further improvements, SCAN-2.1 with CAPSE-2 (Chapter 11) now follows. The Chart lists the stages of development of SCAN, from PSE-7 to SCAN version 2.1.

Chart. The development of PSE into SCAN

PSE-7&8, US/UK and IPSS, 1972/3	CATEGO-1&2
PSE-9, 1974	CATEGO-3&4
Prototype SCAN	1983
SCAN-0, used in field trials;	*1988*
PSE-10.0	CATEGO-5D
Item Group Checklist (ICG)	
Clinical History Schedule (CHS)	
SCAN-1, incorporating experience from field trials	
and early DCR for ICD-10;	*1992*
PSE-10.1	CATEGO-5
IGC-1	CAPSE-1
CHS-1	
SCAN-2.0, incorporating late DCR and DSM-IV;	*1994*
SCAN-2.1, further developed;	*1998*
PSE-10.2	CAPSE-2
ICG-2	
CHS-2	

Note: Several versions of the PSE, SCAN and their computer programs are mentioned in this manual. The chart shows the sequence of development.

Although these changes have altered the scope and complexity of SCAN, its continuity with PSE principles and tradition has been preserved. PSE-9 remained in use in projects covering a wide spectrum of problems, as witnessed by papers published in the British Journal of Psychiatry during 1995 (see Appendix 2.1).

Plan of the book

Chapters 4 to 7 describe in more detail the principles of SCAN using examples from SCAN-2. Chapter 3 summarises the aims of SCAN, defines the way the main technical terms are used and describes the structure of SCAN. The heart of the matter, the Glossary and method of interview, are described in Chapter 4. Chapter 5 is concerned with the problems of translation, Chapter 6 with technical aspects of measurement and Chapter 7 (based on these principles) with training.

Chapter 8 deals with the field trials of SCAN-0, on the basis of which SCAN-1 was developed. The computerised algorithms for early drafts of ICD-10, based on version 1, and the development of the computer-assisted version of the interview, CAPSE-1, are described in Chapter 9. Chapters 10 and 11 are concerned with the equivalent developments for SCAN-2 and CAPSE-2. In so far as it is possible to look forward, the position of SCAN at the beginning of 1998 and its future into the next century are considered by the editors in Chapter 12.

Appendix 2.1

References to PSE-9 in papers published in the *British Journal of Psychiatry*, January to December 1995

Almeida O. P., Howard R. J., Levy R. and David S. D. (1995) Psychotic states arising in late life (late paraphrenia). Psychopathology and nosology. *British Journal of Psychiatry*, 166: 205–14.

Almeida O. P., Howard R. J., Levy R. and David S. D. (1995) Psychotic states arising in late life (late paraphrenia). The role of risk factors. *British Journal of Psychiatry*, 166: 215–28.

Daly I., Webb M. and Kaliszer M. (1995) First admission study of mania, 1975–1981. *British Journal of Psychiatry*, 167: 463–8.

David A., Os J., Jones P., Harvey I., Foerster A. and Fahy T. (1995) Insight and psychotic illness – cross-sectional and longitudinal associations. *British Journal of Psychiatry*, 167: 621–8.

Farmer A., Jones I., Hillier J., LLewelyn M., Borysiewicz L. and Smith A. (1995) Neuraesthenia revisited: ICD-10 and DSM-III-R psychiatric syndromes in chronic fatigue patients and comparison subjects. *British Journal of Psychiatry*, 167: 503–6.

Ferdinand R. F., van der Reijden M., Verhulst F. C., Nienhuis F. J. and Giel R. (1995) Assessment of the prevalence of psychiatric disorder in young adults. *British Journal of Psychiatry*, 166: 480–8.

Gater R. A., Kind P. and Gudex C. (1995) Quality of life in liaison psychiatry. A comparison of patient and clinician assessment. *British Journal of Psychiatry*, 166: 515–20.

Hamid W. A., Wykes T. and Stansfeld S. (1995) The social disablement of men in hostels for homeless people. 1. Reliability and prevalence. *British Journal of Psychiatry*, 166: 809–12.

Hauff E. and Vaglum, P. (1995) Organised violence and the stress of exile. Predictors of mental health in a community cohort of Vietnamese refugees three years after resettlement. *British Journal of Psychiatry*, 166: 360–7.

Hickling F. W. and Rodgers-Johnson P. (1995) The incidence of first contact schizophrenia in Jamaica. *British Journal of Psychiatry*, 167: 193–6.

Hollis C. (1995) Child and adolescent (juvenile onset) schizophrenia. A case control study of premorbid developmental impairments. *British Journal of Psychiatry*, 166: 489–95.

Lawrie S. M., Ingle G. T., Santosh C. G., Rogers A. C., Rimmington J. E., Naidu K. P., Best J. J. K., O'Carroll R. E., Goodwin G. M., Ebmeier K. P. and Johnstone E. C. (1995) MRI and single photon emission tomography in treatment-responsive and treatment-resistant schizophrenia. *British Journal of Psychiatry* 167: 202–10.

Leenstra A. S., Ormel J. and Giel R. (1995) Positive life change and recovery from depression and anxiety. A three-stage longitudinal study of primary care attenders. *British Journal of Psychiatry*, 166: 333–43.

Mason P., Harrison G., Glazebrook C., Medley I., Dalkin T. and Croudace T. (1995) Characteristics of outcome in schizophrenia at 13 years. *British Journal of Psychiatry*, 167: 596–603.

McGilchrist I. and Cutting J. (1995) Somatic delusions in schizophrenia and the affective psychoses. *British Journal of Psychiatry*, 167: 350–61.

Mellors J. D. C., Quinn M. P. and Ron M. A. (1995) Psychotic and depressive symptoms in Parkinson's disease. A study of the growth hormone response to apomorphine. *British Journal of Psychiatry*, 167: 522–6.

Murray D., Cox J. L., Chapman G. and Jones P. (1995) Childbirth. Life event or start of a long-term difficulty? Further data from the Stoke-on-Trent controlled study of postnatal depression. *British Journal of Psychiatry*, 166: 595–600.

Ohaeri J. U., Adeyinka A. O., Enyidah S. N. and Osuntokun B. O. (1995) Schizophrenic and manic brains in Nigerians.

Computerised tomography findings. *British Journal of Psychiatry*, 166: 496–500.

Oldehinkel A. J. and Giel R. (1995) Time trends in the case-based incidence of schizophrenia. *British Journal of Psychiatry*, 167: 777–82.

Os J., Fahy T. A., Jones P., Harvey I., Lewis S., Williams M., Toone B. and Murray R. (1995) Increased intracerebralcerebrospinal fluid spaces predict unemployment and negative symptoms in psychotic illness. A prospective study. *British Journal of Psychiatry*, 166: 750–8.

Susser E., Varma V. K., Malhotra S., Conover S. and Amador X. F. (1995) Delineation of acute and transient psychotic disorders in a developing country setting. *British Journal of Psychiatry*, 167: 216–19.

Telles C., Karno M., Mintz J., Paz G., Arias M., Tucker D. and Lopez S. (1995) Immigrant families coping with schizophrenia. Behavioural intervention v. case management with low-income Spanish-speaking population. *British Journal of Psychiatry*, 167: 473–9.

Wilkinson G., Piccinelli M., Falloon I., Krekorian H. and McLees S. (1995) An evaluation of community-based care for people with long-term mental illness. *British Journal of Psychiatry*, 167: 26–37.

References

Bebbington P. E., Hurry J., Tennant C., Sturt E. and Wing J. K. (1981) Epidemiology of mental disorders in Camberwell. *Psychological Medicine*, 11: 561–80.

Brugha T. S., Wing J. K., Brewin C. R., MacCarthy B., Mangen S., Lesage A. and Mumford J. (1988) The problems of people in long-term psychiatric day-care. An introduction to the Camberwell High Contact Survey. *Psychological Medicine*, 18: 443–56.

Composite International Diagnostic Interview (1995) Washington: WHO and American Psychiatric Press.

Cooper J. E., Copeland J. R. M., Brown G. W., Harris T. and Gourlay J. (1977) Further studies on interviewer training and inter-rater reliability of the PSE. *Psychological Medicine*, 7: 517–23.

Cooper J. E., Kendell R. E., Gurland B. J., Sharpe L., Copeland J. R. M. and Simon R. (1972) *Psychiatric diagnosis in New York and London*. London: Oxford University Press.

Cooper J. E. and McKenzie S. (1981) The rapid prediction of low scores on a standardized psychiatric interview (PSE). In: Wing J. K., Bebbington P. and Robins L. N. (eds.) *What is a case?* London: Grant McIntyre.

Dean C., Surtees P. G. and Sashidharan S. P. (1983) Comparison of research diagnostic systems in an Edinburgh community sample. *British Journal of Psychiatry*, 142: 247–56.

Foulds G. A. (1965) *Personality and personal illness*. London: Tavistock.

Henderson S., Duncan-Jones P., Byrne D. G., Scott R. and Adcock S. (1979) Psychiatric disorder in Canberra. A standardized study of prevalence. *Acta Psychiatrica Scandinavica*, 60: 355–74.

Huxley P., Raval H., Korer J. and Jacob C. (1989) Psychiatric morbidity in the clients of social workers. Clinical outcome. *Psychological Medicine*, 19: 189–98.

International Personality Disorder Examination (1992) Geneva: WHO.

Jablensky A., Sartorius N., Hirschfeld R. and Pardes H. (1983) Diagnosis and classification of mental disorders and alcohol- and drug-related problems. A research agenda for the 1980s. *Psychological Medicine*, 13: 907–21.

Kendell R. R., Everitt B., Cooper J. E., Sartorius N. and David M.E. (1968) Reliability of the PSE. *Social Psychiatry*, 3: 123–9.

Knights A., Hirsch S. R. and Platt S. D. (1980) Clinical change as a function of brief admission to hospital in a controlled study using the PSE. *British Journal of Psychiatry*, 137: 170–80.

Kreitman N. (1961) The reliability of psychiatric diagnosis. *Journal of Mental Science* 107: 876–86.

Lehtinen V., Lindholm T., Veijola J. and Väisänen E. (1990) The prevalence of PSE-CATEGO disorders in a Finnish adult population cohort. *Social Psychiatry and Psychiatric Epidemiology*, 25: 187–92.

Lesage A. D., Cyr M. and Toupin J. (1991) Reliable use of the PSE by psychiatric nurses of psychotic and non-psychotic patients. *Acta Psychiatrica*, 83: 121–4.

Lorr M. (ed.), (1996) *Explorations in typing psychotics*. London and New York: Pergamon.

Luria R. E. and Berry R. (1979) Reliability and descriptive validity of the PSE syndromes. *Archives of General Psychiatry*, 36: 1187–95.

Luria R. E. and McHugh P. R. (1974) Reliability and clinical utility of the Wing PSE. *Archives of General Psychiatry*, 30: 866–71.

McGuffin P., Katz R. and Aldrich J. (1986) Past and present state examination. The assessment of 'lifetime ever' psychopathology. *Psychological Medicine*, 16: 461–6.

O'Connor N. (1968) The origins of the Medical Research Council Social Psychiatry Unit. In: Shepherd M. and Davies D. L. (eds.) *Studies in psychiatry*. London: Oxford University Press.

Okasha A. and Ashour A. (1981) Psycho-demographic study of anxiety in Egypt. The PSE in its Arabic version. *British Journal of Psychiatry*, 139: 70–3.

Orley J. and Wing J. K. (1979) Psychiatric disorders in two African villages. *Archives of General Psychiatry*, 36: 513–20.

Rogers B. and Mann S. A. (1986) The reliability and validity of PSE assessments by lay interviewers. A national population survey. *Psychological Medicine*, 16: 689–700.

Rose G. (1992) *The strategy of preventive medicine*. Oxford University Press.

Sturt E. (1981) Hierarchical patterns in the distribution of psychiatric symptoms. *Psychological Medicine*, 11: 783–94.

Tress K. H., Bellenis C., Brownlow J. H., Livingston G. and Leff J. P. (1987) The PSE change rating scale. *British Journal of Psychiatry*, 150: 201–7.

Urwin P. and Gibbons J. L. (1979) Psychiatric diagnosis in self poisoning patients. *Psychological Medicine*, 9: 501–7.

Venables P. H. (1957) A short scale for 'activity-withdrawal' in schizophrenics. *Journal of Mental Science*, 103: 197–9.

Venables P. H. and O'Connor N. (1959) A short scale for rating paranoid schizophrenia. *Journal of Mental Science*, 105: 815–18.

Venables P. H. and Wing J. K. (1962) Level of arousal and the subclassification of schizophrenia. *Archives of General Psychiatry*, 7: 114–19.

Wing J. K. (1959) The measurement of behaviour in chronic schizophrenia. *Acta Psychiatrica et Neurologica*, 35: 245–54.

Wing J. K. (1961) A simple and reliable subclassification of chronic schizophrenia. *Journal of Mental Science*, 107: 862–75.

Wing J. K. (1962) Institutionalism in mental hospitals. *Journal of Social and Clinical Psychology*, 1: 38–51.

Wing J. K. (1976) A technique for studying psychiatric morbidity in inpatient and out-patient series and in general population samples. *Psychological Medicine*, 6: 665–71.

Wing J. K. (1983) Use and misuse of the PSE. *British Journal of Psychiatry*, 143: 111–17.

Wing J. K. (1988) Comments on the long term outcome of schizophrenia. *Schizophrenia Bulletin*, 14: 669–72.

Wing J. K. (1994) Relevance of psychiatric epidemiology to clinical psychiatry. *International Review of Psychiatry*, 6: 259–64.

Wing J. K. (1995) SCAN and the PSE tradition (1995). *Social Psychiatry and Psychiatric Epidemiology*, 31: 50–4.

Wing J. K., Bebbington P. E. and Robins L. N. (1981) Theory testing in psychiatric epidemiology. In: Wing J. K., Bebbington P. E. and Robins

L. N. (eds.) What is a case? The problem of definition in psychiatric community surveys. London: Grant McIntyre.

Wing J. K., Birley J. L. T., Cooper J. E., Graham P. and Isaacs A. D. (1967) Reliability of a procedure for measuring and classifying 'present psychiatric stata'. *British Journal of Psychiatry*, 113: 499–515.

Wing J. K., Babor T., Brugha T., Burke J., Cooper J., Giel R., Jablensky A., Regier D. and Sartorius N. (1990) SCAN: Schedules for clinical assessment in neuropsychiatry. *Archives of General Psychiatry*, 47: 589–93.

Wing J. K., Cooper J. E. and Sartorius N. (1974) *The description and classification of psychiatric symptoms. An instruction manual for the PSE and CATEGO system.* London: Cambridge University Press.

Wing J. K. and Hailey A H. (eds.) (1972) *Evaluating a community psychiatric service. The Camberwell Register 1964–1971.* London: Oxford University Press.

Wing J. K., Nixon J. M., von Cranach M. and Strauss A. (1980) Further developments of the PSE and CATEGO system. In: Bartko J. J. and Gulbinat W. (eds.) *Multivariate statistical methodologies used in the IPSS*, chapter 4, pp. 46–54. Mental Health Service System Reports. Rockville: ADAMHA.

Wing J. K., Mann S. A., Leff J. P. and Nixon J. M. (1978) The concept of a 'case' in psychiatric population surveys. *Psychological Medicine*, 8: 203–17.

Wing J. K., Nixon J. M., Mann S. A. and Leff J. P. (1977) Reliability of the PSE (ninth edition) used in a population survey. *Psychological Medicine*, 7: 505–16.

Wittenborn J. R. (1955) *Wittenborn Psychiatric Rating Scales.* New York: Psychological Corporation.

World Health Organization (1973) *The international pilot study of schizophrenia.* Geneva: WHO.

World Health Organization (1979) *Schizophrenia. An international follow-up study.* Geneva: WHO.

World Health Organization (1990) *International classification of diseases*, tenth edition, Geneva: WHO.

3 Aims and structure of SCAN

J. K. Wing

Three aims in one

The aim of SCAN can be stated very simply, in one sentence. It is to provide comprehensive, accurate and technically specifiable means of describing and classifying clinical phenomena, in order to make comparisons. Making comparisons is at the heart of all clinical, educational and scientific activities. Even making a single assessment using SCAN provides the opportunity to make comparisons with other patients known to the same clinician. Every interview and every prescription can be seen as a clinical experiment.

The first, clinical, aim is to promote high-quality clinical observation. PSE-10 is designed to allow a comparison of the respondent's experiences and behaviour against the examiner's Glossary-defined concepts, by a process of controlled clinical cross-examination. The resulting symptom profiles, scores and rule-based categories of disorder, can be compared with each other wherever in the world they are produced, and used for clinical audit, needs assessment and monitoring of progress of individual respondents.

The second aim, educational and developmental, is to improve clinical concepts by teaching a common clinical language. This makes it feasible to compare, and learn from, the usage of different clinical schools. It is not necessary to agree with a common standard of reference to appreciate its value as a basis for communication and comparison. Different clinical schools of thought do exist and are taught. Comparison between them by means of a common standard of reference provides a basis for informed development.

The third, scientific, aim is to accelerate the accumulation of knowledge. Using standard technical procedures in research projects makes the results more precise and comparable, thus leading to more rapid agreement on useful theoretical lines for further research. This is true of all types of scientific research – biological, epidemiological and psychosocial.

The three aims together facilitate the accumulation of knowledge for clinical purposes of all kinds, including primary, secondary and tertiary prevention and high quality health-service management and planning. SCAN itself will benefit, both from the comparisons it has supported and from the results of the work it has facilitated. New item-concepts will be added and old ones improved. But modifications should be made in carefully designed stages, following periods of experience long enough to provide a substantial basis for change. This is how SCAN has developed so far.

SCAN terminology

SCAN covers aspects of experience or behaviour that are common among people referred for a specialist psychiatric opinion. Each aspect is allocated an item in the SCAN text, with a unique item-number and item-name. The corresponding definitions are listed in the Glossary (Chapter 4) in numerical order. 'Items' represent subjectively described 'symptoms' or 'signs' observed in behaviour. Symptoms and signs are sometimes referred to as 'phenomena'.

These terms might suggest that the items are linked to theories of cause or pathology, and therefore that SCAN items might represent symptoms and signs of diseases. Such hypotheses are for test, they are not assertions. A central principle is that phenomena are rated on their own merits, irrespective of any theory about the way they cluster, their causes or their psychosocial or biological nature. It is only in this way that a comprehensive clinical picture can be obtained, on which classifying and/or dimensional rules of various kinds can operate. No particular set of rules should be allowed to influence decisions as to whether any symptom or sign is present. Terms like 'neurotic', 'affective', 'psychotic' and 'organic' are used descriptively, in the same spirit. The interviewing style that achieves this is also described in Chapter 4.

In some items, the examiner can make an attribution about pathology or etiology or relationship to other phenomena, but these are clinical judgements required by rule-based diagnostic systems such as ICD-10, not specifications by the SCAN system. The terminology of symptoms and signs is used for convenience only.

Thus the SCAN text is truly 'bottom-up', in the sense that it provides a means of gathering data according to the Glossary definitions, independently of the type of 'top-down' classification that might be applied. These data can be used to provide profiles and scores of many different kinds. SCAN, like its predecessors, is not simply, or even primarily, 'a diagnostic instrument', although its database is broad enough to allow the application of a range of diagnostic algorithms, including those of the ICD and DSM.

Some terms commonly used in SCAN are described in more detail below. Certain of them are used with a strictly limited meaning and it is important to understand the reasons why.

Item

The numbered 'items' are the simplest structures in SCAN. Clinical items represent subjective experiences or observed behaviours that are differentially defined in the Glossary. Each has an 'item concept' and should only be rated according to this definition. It is not necessary for the interviewer to agree with the definition to use it in order to make comparisons.

Conventionally, such items are called 'symptoms' or 'signs', the implication being that they are manifestations of some underlying cause. All these terms are used descriptively, with the same connotation as 'item'. Each item is rated on its own merits, irrespective of any theoretical relationships to other items or to putative shared causes. Diagnostic theories – for example, preconceived ideas as to how items should cluster together – must not be allowed to influence ratings.

Trait

Traits have been present more or less throughout the respondent's adult life, with no recent exacerbation or 'onset'. They are rated separately from symptoms in SCAN-1, but with optional attributional rating at item level in SCAN versions 2.0 and 2.1.

Item group

Every clinical item in SCAN has its place in an 'Item Group', composed of items of roughly similar type. Some of these can be rated separately in an Item Group Checklist, in order to rate episodes from case-records. The others are less suitable for retrospective rating. However, the constituent PSE-10 item ratings of all Item Groups can be summed to give Item Group scores and profiles for each respondent.

Disorder

'Disorder' is a rule-based construct, as described, for example, in the Diagnostic Criteria for Research (DCR) of ICD-10 (see page 1, Chapter 1).

Diagnosis

'Diagnosis' is not a term that is much used in SCAN or ICD-10 terminology. This is partly to avoid influencing the way items are rated, since the presence and severity of a symptom or behaviour should be assessed on its own specific merits and not on prior expectation of how it 'ought' to cluster with others. Even the use of Sections, Item Groups and Scores based on notional 'symptom types' does not contradict the basic principle that all items are rated individually, irrespective of the presence or absence of any other.

The categories derived by the computer algorithms (Chapters 9 and 11) depend: (a) on the symptom ratings and the attributions of cause or pathology made by the interviewer; (b) on the rules of ICD-10–DCR (or other such system). SCAN is a tool; it cannot make a diagnosis. Only the user of the tool can determine whether the quality of the data-set collected in a particular case, and the computerised classification based on it, means anything in diagnostic terms. The clinical user must decide whether to accept or reject the category or categories produced by the application of SCAN. In some cases, e.g. in research studies under strictly specified conditions, this may be automatic. But the interviewer should always know whether the interview is sufficiently adequate to allow a diagnosis based on it to be taken seriously. There is provision in the Clinical History Schedule for writing in an independent clinical diagnosis. This should always be entered in order to allow the comparison.

The structure of SCAN

SCAN may be defined as a set of instruments aimed at assessing, measuring and classifying the psychopathology and behaviour associated with the major psychiatric disorders of adult life. The components needed to achieve the aims are the SCAN tools:

- The SCAN-2.1 manual, comprising

  - The Present State Examination, tenth edition (PSE-10)
  - The Item Group Checklist (IGC), Section 26,
  - The Clinical History Schedule (CHS), Section 27,

- The SCAN Glossary

- The CAPSE-2 computer application
- The SCAN training material
- The SCAN reference manual

The SCAN interview manual, version 2.1

PSE-10

The tenth edition of the PSE is the largest part of the SCAN manual, taking up the first 25 sections of SCAN-2. These are listed at Appendix 3.1. Each section is devoted to a particular type of symptom or sign or other clinical feature. The sections cover the symptoms and signs of disorders in subchapters F0–F5 of ICD-10, and their equivalents in DSM-III-R and DSM-IV.

F0   Organic, including symptomatic, mental disorders
F1   Mental and behavioural disorders due to psychoactive substance use
F2   Schizophrenia, schizotypal and delusional disorders
F3   Mood (affective) disorders
F4   Neurotic, stress-related and somatoform disorders
F50–51   Eating disorders; Non-organic sleep disorders

Some sections have optional checklists attached, covering items related to disorders that require specific time relationships, for example to psychosocial trauma, as in the stress and adjustment disorders. Other checklists allow a more extended list of items to be rated than is provided in the main text; for example the checklist for Persistent Depressive States, Dysthymia.

The main headings in subchapter F6 of ICD-10, for personality disorders, are included as a list in the CHS, for direct rating. The International Personality Disorder Examination, developed under the auspices of WHO and ADAMHA, is recommended for use in association with SCAN if a full assessment is required. Subchapters F7 (mental retardation), F8 (development disorders), and F9 (disorders with an onset in childhood), are also not covered in detail, since the interview format is not generally suited to eliciting their problems. However, provision is made for direct rating in the CHS.

When people with F6–F9 disorders do suffer from the problems listed in F0–F5 as well and can be interviewed using the PSE, some of the ratings will be relevant to their main condition. Behavioural problems common to disorders in the autistic spectrum (F84.0, F84.1) are covered because, in the form known as Asperger's syndrome, those afflicted are often able to take part in the examination and enjoy doing so. However, disorders in F7–9 will not be adequately covered unless a developmental history is taken and other instruments are used as well.

Item Group Checklist: Section 26

The Item Group Checklist (IGC) provides a simple means of rating information obtained only from case-records and/or informants other than the respondent. The IGs are not diagnostic syndromes; they cannot be translated directly into ICD-10 disorders, but will be processed by a version of the CAPSE program developed from the one that is applied to data from PSE-10. The resulting classification will be approximate compared with that from PSE-10 but provide a useful supplement to PSE information, and substitute in situations where the PSE cannot be fully completed.

The 40 Item Groups included in the checklist cover disorders in subchapters F2 (psychoses), F3 (affective disorders) and F40–42 (neuroses) of ICD-10. Disorders in subchapters F0 (cognitive impairment), F1 (substance use disorders), F43–45 (stress, dissociative and somatoform disorders) and F5 (appetite and sleep disorders and sexual dysfunctions), which are difficult to rate without interviewing or examining the respondent, are not included. It may occasionally be appropriate (particularly for the eating and substance use disorders) to rate the full PSE-10 from case-records or an informant.

Users of the IGC must have been trained in the use of the PSE and its Glossary, and be completely familiar with the structure of SCAN.

This provides a substantial degree of operationalisation for rating IGs, each of which is composed of designated PSE-10 items.

There are three main indications for using the IGC:

1 When the Respondent can provide information about present state but is unable or unwilling to remember or describe accurately the events or symptoms of a previous episode. In such a case, the previous period (see Chapter 6) is chosen and dated in the same way as for the PSE. However, it is not necessary, for most purposes, to use IGC to rate a past episode if the symptoms then were very similar to those in the present state.

2 When an interview with the respondent is impossible. The period/s chosen will depend on a clinical judgement as to which will most adequately cover the history. Often there will be an opportunity to observe behaviour, speech and affect on examination, even when an interview is impossible.

3 For use in research projects that require the maximum use of information in case-records. Even when two PSEs have been completed, extra IGCs can be processed separately as a supplement to the routine package.

Section 27. Clinical History Schedule

The CHS supplements the information collected in PSE-10 and the IGC by providing an opportunity to check or enter data relevant to the broader clinical and social history, and also to rate the presence or absence of disorders in subchapters F6–F9 of ICD-10.

Several of the items involve a rating of performance relative to local expectation; a judgement that can only be made by someone familiar with the local culture and environment. The subsections of the CHS are listed in Appendix 3.1.

The CHS is optional, but is recommended because of the opportunity it offers to match the information against data recorded elsewhere in SCAN. A simple statistical package will be provided with the computer software (see Chapter 11) which will enable the user, after collecting a series of cases, to examine profiles of diagnoses or scores against age, sex, personality, disablement, physical illness etc. Comorbidity, for example, is a prominent feature of mental illness, as Figures 1–8 in Chapter 8 illustrate.

Data recording

The SCAN examination serves to structure the collection of clinical information, which is covered by rating boxes in the SCAN schedule itself, in fixed-format SCAN Coding Booklets, free-format Coding Pads, or directly into a computer. This last method is particularly convenient because the data can be analysed as soon as the interview is complete, and also because the Glossary definitions can be brought to the screen for easy reference. Chapters 9 and 11 deal with methods of data entry and with the range of programs available.

Appendix 3.1   List of contents: SCAN-2.1

Present State Examination 10.2: Part One

Section 0

Introduction to SCAN
Face sheet
Sociodemographic information

Section 1

Beginning the interview: contingencies
Introductions and overview of clinical problems
Selection of episodes
Medication
Psychosocial interventions
Other aspects of clinical history
Rating scale I
Optional etiology attribution scale

Section 2

Somatoform and dissociative symptoms
Dissociative symptoms

Section 3

Worrying, tension etc.

Section 4

Panic, anxiety and phobias

Section 5

Obsessional symptoms

Section 6

Depressed mood and ideation
Checklist: Dysthymia
Checklist: Recurrent brief depressive disorder

Section 7

Thinking, concentration, energy, interests

Section 8

Bodily functions

Section 9

Eating disorders

Section 10

Expansive mood and ideation
Checklist: Cyclothymia

Section 11

Use of alcohol

Section 12

Use of psychoactive substances other than alcohol
Checklists: other drugs
Tobacco use

Section 13

Interferences and attributions for Part One

Stress and adjustment disorders
Adequacy of interview
Item level Attributional Rating Scale

Section 14

Screen for Part Two

Present State Examination 10.2: Part Two

Section 15

Language problems at examination
Rating scale II

Section 16

Perceptual disorders other than hallucinations

Section 17

Hallucinations

Section 18

Experiences of disorder of thought and replacement of will

Section 19

Delusions

Section 20

Further information for classification of Part Two disorders
Checklists: Acute psychosis
                Induced psychotic disorder
                Schizotypal disorder
                Simple schizophrenia
Interferences and attributions for Part Two
Psychosocial factors influencing manifestation of symptoms
Negative syndrome and items
Adequacy of interview

Section 21

Cognitive impairment and decline
Aetiology of cognitive impairment
Checklist: Mild cognitive disorder

Section 22

Rating scale III
Motor and behavioural items

Section 23

Affect

Section 24

Speech abnormalities
Insight and adequacy of information

Section 25

Autistic Spectrum Checklist

Item Group Checklist (IGC)

Section 26

Rating scale IV
Introduction
IG1 (nervous tension) to IG40 (catatonic behaviour)
Adequacy of information in IGC

Clinical History Schedule

Section 27

Introduction
Childhood and education
Intellectual level
Social roles and performance
Overall social handicap
Disorders of adult personality and behaviour
Quality of data recorded in SCAN
Overall clinical diagnoses

4 The SCAN Glossary and principles of the interview

J. K. Wing

Introduction

Both the limitations and the advantages of SCAN stem from the nature of the problems it attempts to solve. These problems are not specific to psychiatry but they are more obvious and more complex than many of those met elsewhere in medicine, largely because the most characteristic symptoms are subjective; known only because a person describes them. Observable signs do exist, such as autonomic arousal in someone describing a subjective feeling of anxiety, or evidence of concomitant activity in the cortex while describing auditory hallucinations. But the reported experience is often the only evidence available. The first and most basic problem, therefore, is to decide whether a symptom is present or absent. The second problem, an extension of the first, is to assess clinical severity.

In many cases, particularly during an acute attack, both decisions are relatively simple because the symptom is clearly present in severe degree. In others, the experience described is so rare that, unless there is evidence to the contrary (e.g. contacts with medical textbooks or with people who talk about the experience, together with possible reasons for dissimulation) an accurate description is adequate to establish its presence, if not its severity. Some first-rank symptoms are of this type. Other symptoms, such as anxiety and depression, are very common in mild degree. Should they nevertheless be rated as present, if there is no reason to doubt the description, even though they are accompanied by only trivial interference with occupational or personal functioning? Such decisions are of great importance in general practice or a general population survey.

No selection of symptoms, and no set of definitions, will satisfy everybody. Nor should they. Karl Koehler (1979) observed that the only interesting question in such circumstances is whether divergent views about particular symptoms can be specified. If not, discussion may be fascinating but cannot reach conclusions. There is a risk in relying only on criteria that are communicable and can be checked

(Berner et al., 1980; Berner and Kuffele, 1982), since concepts that cannot be defined may have value when used by percipient clinicians who are nevertheless unable to provide a definition for general use. But until they are more precisely specified they cannot be understood and reliably used for comparative purposes.

The presence or absence of a symptom is determined in SCAN solely by using the technique of interviewing known as clinical cross-examination, in which interviewer and respondent engage in a process of matching the experience described against the differential definitions provided in the Glossary.

Severity is defined in two ways; by providing rating scales appropriate to the type of symptom or other item, and by providing examples of specific points on the severity scale as part of the Glossary definition of individual items. For example, the presence of many neurotic symptoms is determined by the extent to which they are out of the conscious control of the respondent, out of proportion to circumstances, and accompanied by an unpleasant affect. Each criterion contributes to the decision, but none is used alone. If 'worrying', for example, is appropriate to the circumstances but out of voluntary control and experienced as painful in itself, it is present; the severity is then determined by the intensity of the disturbance of will and emotion, together with duration and frequency during a given time period. Social causes of such problems are not taken into account in the rating (they should be rated on other instruments), except in judging the proportionality of the response. However, individual factors affecting the reporting of symptoms, such as degree of stoicism and culturally acceptable ways of expressing the complaint, must necessarily be considered. Technical details of the measurement of severity throughout SCAN are provided in Chapter 6.

Extensive experience has demonstrated that it is possible for virtually all trained clinicians to apply the definitions in the Glossary even if they would not themselves agree with some of them. (There are rare exceptions.) The point of using SCAN is not to ensure uniformity of thought, but to provide a reference system against which to make comparisons for clinical, educational and research purposes.

Structure of the Glossary

The Glossary has been developed from that of PSE-9, in the light of the accumulated experience of users, and expanded to take in the new areas of phenomena. The definitions of equivalent items remain substantially the same, but there has often been some elaboration or clarification and the rating scale has been extended. Information from the text of ICD-10, its Diagnostic Criteria for Research (DCR), and the DSM series, has been incorporated where appropriate. Chiefly, however, the editorial group has relied on the experience of large numbers of users and on the detailed comments of consultants.

The Glossary presents SCAN items in numerical order, by sections. Each section has an introduction that describes how the general principles of definition are applied, or occasionally modified, for that group of symptoms. Sections are clinically based. Statistical analyses produce other arrangements of items that will be useful in determining the psychometric properties of SCAN but are not convenient for interviewing purposes. Nearly all clinical items in PSE-10 contain a brief definition in the interview manual. Those that involve clinical cross-examination are provided with a list of probes to elicit relevant information from the respondent, and instructions for numerical rating. The Glossary definition is usually more detailed and provides reasons for excluding other possible symptoms. Most 'technical' items in SCAN, such as those dealing with dates, causal attributions, predominance of certain symptom types over others, specific time relationships during the course etc, also have an explanatory text (see Chapter 6). The Glossary is therefore not only a dictionary of terms, but a commentary on the way that SCAN should be used. It can be consulted whenever a problem arises that cannot be answered from the SCAN text.

Examples of Glossary definitions

Three PSE-10 items, one common, two rare, will be used to illustrate some of the principles of definition.

3.002: Subjective feeling of nervous tension

The first is 'nervous tension', item 3.002 in the text of PSE-10.2, Section 3. The item is not chosen for illustration because of its clinical significance. It is common in the general population and virtually non-specific for an ICD-10 diagnosis, as are many other Section 3 items (Sturt, 1981). But the basis for definition is similar to that for many symptoms included in the rules for F4 'neurotic' disorders, and is therefore useful for demonstration purposes. The introduction to Section 3 of the Glossary specifies that all the symptoms included can occur alone, or in association with each other, and with or without more specific phenomena such as anxiety or depression. The definition is as follows:

A feeling of inner restlessness or unease expressed in terms such as 'nerves', 'being on edge', 'being keyed up'. Being 'up-tight', or 'wound up', implies a degree of muscular tension as well and the two symptoms commonly coexist.

Nervous tension is a state of arousal that has three basic characteristics of many non-specific and neurotic symptoms – it is unpleasant, not under voluntary control and not fully explicable in situational terms. There is likely to be an exaggerated startle response. Autonomic symptoms (Section 4) may or may not be frankly present; they are not a requirement for the symptom. Nervous tension is not linked to any particular mental content though it often does accompany symptoms such as worry and anxiety, and may appear as a precursor to them.

Differentiation from other symptoms:

Muscular tension (item 3.003) is frequently present but it is not the same symptom and should be rated independently. Nervous tension should be differentiated from anxiety (item 4.023) and anxious foreboding (item 4.024), for which clear-cut autonomic symptoms must be present.

Normal situational nervousness, such as being keyed up before an examination, should be rated 0, not 1.

6.007: Feeling of loss of feeling

The second example is from Section 6, concerned with depressed mood and ideation. 'Feeling of loss of feeling' involves a deficit of emotions, but its definition need not be vague. It was defined originally by German writers, who regarded it as of major significance in the diagnosis of melancholia. 'Die Gefüllosigkeit wird gefült, die Erstarrung empfunden, die Leblosigkeit erlebt' (Bleuler, 1953). This is quoted in the text of the PSE-10 interview: 'The loss of feeling is felt, the numbness perceived, the lifelessness experienced.' The definition in the Glossary is as follows:

The respondents must describe a definite *loss* of the ability to feel emotion, compared with their normal state. They can remember a time, which might have been months or years earlier, when they did have the capacity for feeling. The symptom need not have begun during the period being rated. An example is an elderly depressed woman who can no longer feel the love she had (and says she still has) for her grandchildren. The inability to feel this love causes severe distress.

The symptom is usually associated with depressed mood, particularly if there is chronic apathy. It can also be associated with irritability and with affects such as anxiety. Respondents may also say they are depressed, meaning that an earlier mood of sadness has been replaced by numbness or that the two symptoms are present together.

Differentiation from other symptoms:

This is a subjective complaint and should not be confused with observed 'Blunting of affect' (item 23.012). It is not delusional and it is not lack of insight. On the contrary, it is a realistic description of a state of mind. There is no equivalent 'trait' since the symptom must have an onset.

Section 19: The differential definition of 'delusion'

The third example, from the introduction to Section 19 on delusions, specifies the rules that govern the differential recognition and rating of a 'delusion' during the interaction between interviewer and patient. This introduction is followed by 32 items concerned with particular types of delusion and delusional elaboration.

The Glossary text begins with a reference to definitions for other psychotic symptoms in Sections 16–18 and specifies that respondents with a language or speech problem, including vague or rambling speech pose particular problems, rated in Section 15. Eleven points are made to aid definition.

The first four concern necessary but not sufficient characteristics of a delusion:

1. The belief is described clearly in the respondent's own words, not simply assented to following a leading question.
2. It is held with a basic and compelling subjective conviction, though the degree of certainty may fluctuate or be concealed.
3. It is not susceptible, or only briefly, to modification by experience or evidence that contradicts it; i.e. it is incorrigible.
4. The belief is impossible, incredible or false.

Three kinds of belief may have all the above four characteristics but are not delusional. Each is defined in the text of the Glossary. The headings are:

5. Social, cultural, religious and political beliefs
6. Overvalued ideas
7. Induced delusions

Finally, four types of phenomena usually regarded as delusional are defined:

8.   Delusions based on abnormal affect
9.   Delusional elaboration of 'primary' phenomena.
10. Pathoplastic delusions; true delusions, expressed in a form familiar to members of a defined social group but usually recognised by them as alien to their beliefs.
11. Primary delusions

19.004: Delusions of reference

Item 19.004 is an example of a differential definition for a particular kind of delusion.

Delusions of reference involve an incorrect attribution of significance to people, objects or events that are perceived normally. They are neither hallucinations nor illusions. Delusions of this type may take the form of a sudden conviction that a given set of perceptions refers to the respondent and has a special significance.

Thus what is said may have a double meaning, or someone makes a gesture that may be construed as a deliberate message; e.g. someone crossing their legs may be taken to mean that the respondent is homosexual. The whole neighbourhood may seem to be gossiping about respondents far beyond the bounds of possibility, or they may see references to themselves on the television or in newspapers. Items 19.005–19.011 concern extensions to other situations, e.g. delusional misinterpretation or misidentification.

Differentiation from other symptoms:

The symptom must be differentiated from auditory hallucinations. It is, of course, possible for respondents to have both symptoms but they are not identical. If they answer 'Yes' to a question about hearing 'voices', it may be that they think that people are talking about them, or making remarks intended for them to overhear. If so, it is likely that they are misinterpreting, not hearing voices. Careful questioning should enable the examiner to judge whether one or the other or both symptoms are present.

Principles of the SCAN interview

The principles of the PSE-10 examination have changed very little since the early days of the instrument.

1. The interview is clinically highly structured, although this may not be apparent when a skilled examiner is in action.
2. The approach is bottom-up; that is to say, it is dependent entirely on matching item-concepts carried in the examiner's mind against experiences described by the respondent in response to probing.
3. The decision as to whether a symptom or sign is present is entirely in the hands of the examiner. It does not depend on the respondent saying 'Yes' or otherwise agreeing to a question.
4. The interview is clinically flexible. It can be varied in order to suit the circumstances, which are unique to each occasion of examination. Where and how to start the interview, whether to jump a Section or return to modify one already rated, whether to pass cut-off points and so on, are in the hands of the examiner.

These characteristics are built into the interview with the overriding aim of providing ratings that are the numerical equivalents of high-quality clinical judgements. The method is known as 'clinical cross-examination'.

Clinical cross-examination

Training in the Glossary, and becoming completely familiar with the differential definitions of items, provides the examiner with a system of item-concepts. The respondent, structured by probes from the PSE schedule, describes (with as few prompts as possible) his or her subjective experiences. There follows a process of question and answer that continues until a match between item-concept and description is found or ruled out. (There are, of course, other rating options, as well as present or absent.) An analogous process is used to rate the presence or absence of behavioural signs.

The term 'cross-examination' may sound very legal and formal, but, in fact, respondents usually find the method quite acceptable. They understand that the interviewer is taking their experiences and complaints seriously. It is a collaborative enterprise between two people trying to arrive at a truth.

For example, in the case of the difficult symptom (item 6.007), 'Feeling of loss of feeling' described above, the PSE-10 manual includes suggestions for use when the interviewer reaches the item. These can be modified as necessary in accordance with the flow of answers to previous questions about mood, e.g.:

Sometimes people don't describe sadness or depression as such but say they have lost the ability to feel any emotion at all. They can't feel sad and can't cry. Have you experienced that sort of lack?

Further probes can follow if indicated:

Can you describe it?
What is that like?
When did you last have ordinary feelings of happiness or sadness or other emotions?
How severe . . .?
Have you been free of it at all?

Bleuler's words are quoted in the PSE interview text and a brief definition included: 'This should be a definite loss compared with the normal state but the loss need not have begun during the period under review.'

The interviewer is free to ask as many or as few questions as the context requires. It may happen that the respondent's spontaneous description may provide all that is necessary for decision. In this way, the glossary definition, the suggested form and context of questioning, and the brief definition in the interview text, provide guidance to the examiner as to how to decide, from the respondent's description, whether the symptom is or is not present. The final decision as to whether the respondent's description matches the description in the Glossary is left to the interviewer's judgement.

References

Berner P., Gabriel E. and Schanda H. (1980) Non-schizophrenic paranoid syndromes, *Schizophrenia Bulletin*, 6: 627–32.

Berner P. and Kufferle B. (1982) British phenomenological and psycho-pathological concepts. A comparative review. *British Journal of Psychiatry*, 140: 558–65.

Bleuler E. (1953) *Lehrbuch der Psychiatrie*. Fünfzehnte Auflage neubear-beitet von Bleuler M., s 233. Heidelberg: Springer-Verlag.

Koehler K. (1979) First rank symptoms of schizophrenia. Questions concerning clinical boundaries. *British Journal of Psychiatry* 134: 236–49.

Sturt E. (1981) Hierarchical patterns in the distribution of psychiatric symptoms. *Psychological Medicine*, 11: 783–94.

5   SCAN translation

N. Sartorius

Introduction

Comparisons of the results of research undertaken in varied cultural settings can be misleading unless comparable methods have been used to collect the data. Depending on the nature of the text, the differences in meaning may be easy or difficult to detect. For example, redundancy in describing a particular event may help to convey meaning and facts correctly in spite of a non-equivalence in meaning of particular passages, phrases or words in the translated version. In questionnaires and standardised assessment instruments, however, non-equivalence can seriously distort results. Prince and Mombour (1967), for example, assigned 80 bilingual subjects randomly to two groups. The first group was given half of the Langner 22 item questionnaire (at that time used for screening purposes) in English, followed by the other half in French. The second group was given the questionnaire with the French half first and the English second. In four of the 22 items the frequency of positive answers differed significantly between the two languages, even though they have similar structure and syntax, and share a significant number of words. In a more recent study, Pichot and colleagues (1991, personal communication) compared the results obtained when the QD2 instrument – a self-report questionnaire containing items usually found in depressive illness – was given in Arabic and French to two groups of bilingual subjects. There was a significant difference between the two language versions on 24 items, all but two of which were scored higher in French. This was true for both male and female respondents. It is obvious that the danger of distortion is much larger if the languages belong to different families and the subjects have very different cultural backgrounds.

Tests of equivalence are also important when an instrument is applied to groups belonging to culturally or socially very distinct groups, although speaking the same language. The risk of distortion is lower with semi-standardised instruments applied by well-trained interviewers conversant with the culture and the languages in which the instrument is applied, than when a fully standardised instrument is used. Nevertheless the risk exists and should be borne in mind in testing the instrument and interpreting the results.

Several aspects of equivalence should be considered when comparing different language versions of a clinical instrument. For example, there may be equivalence of the common meaning of a term, but no equivalence with respect to the use of that word to name a symptom. A full assessment requires examination of three aspects: semantic, conceptual and technical equivalence.

Semantic equivalence

Semantic equivalence includes both the denotative and the connotative aspects of words used in instruments and interviews. The denotation of words (their cognitive meaning) can be examined using dictionary definitions. It relies mainly on linguistic analysis. The connotation of words refers to their emotional meaning and can be studied using the results of anthropological analyses and techniques such as Osgood's semantic differential (1952) and Kelly's repertory grid (1955).

Denotations of words, and to an extent their connotations, can also be studied by comparison of semantic space. Synonyms of a word describe the semantic space it occupies: an equivalent word in another language would occupy a similar semantic space, and most such synonyms would also have a direct counterpart in the other language.

The process of examining semantic space can be time consuming, and is rarely undertaken for all the terms used in a questionnaire. The use of bilingual groups and focus groups (see below) can help identify terms for which semantic equivalence should be examined. In the question, 'Do you avoid . . . (a particular situation)?', for example, the word 'avoid' would be a candidate for such an examination. If the translation were from English into French, this would proceed as follows.

'Avoid', in a medium-size dictionary, has the following correspondences in French, for the varied situations in which it is used:

éviter	échapper	esquiver	se soustraire
frauder	fuir	se dispenser	

The word 'éviter', according to the dictionary, is closest to the act of avoiding a person or a situation. Its meaning can be translated into English by:

avoid   dodge   steer clear of
duck   evade   prevent

The translation of the other words describing 'avoid' in French can be rendered into English by:

échapper	escape, get away from, elude
esquiver	sidestep, dodge
se soustraire	shirk, get out
frauder	shirk, cheat, elude
fuir	fly, run away,
se dispenser	liberate, shirk, get rid of.

The translation of the other words describing 'éviter' in French can be rendered in English by:

dodge	esquiver, détour
steer clear of	éviter, fuir, s'abstenir
duck	esquiver un coup
evade	esquiver, éviter, échapper, se dérober, se soustraire, contourner, frauder
prevent	empécher, éviter.

This comparison of two English and two French sets of near synonyms shows that the word 'éviter', by its synonyms, matches the word 'avoid' in the sense defined by the context of the question. Some terms (such as 'se dérober', 'contourner', 'empécher') do not have an exactly corresponding term in the English series. It is also probable that the translation of 'avoid' by 'éviter' is correct for the sentence cited, but also that 'éviter' would not necessarily have to be translated by 'avoid' if the original were French and the target language English.

The choice of synonyms depends on the linguistic context. In spoken language some synonyms will appear mostly in a context determined by the social class, closeness and shared memories and traditions of the speakers. In professional groups belonging to the same discipline, the choice of synonyms may also be firmly determined. Deviation from the customary choice of synonyms can lead to misunderstanding and emotional tension.

It is occasionally necessary, and often useful, to combine a study of the connotation and denotation of words with consideration of the etymology of a clinical word in different languages. An analysis of the word 'anxiety', for example, provides valuable hints for the choice of items to be included in an instrument (Sartorius, 1990).

In Slavic languages, for example, notions of 'anxiety' and 'fear' are clearly separate. The word for 'fear' is close to that for passion, and its root is linked to anger, trepidation and words for beating and battle. There is a close relationship between the family of words for fear and the word 'strava' (meaning terror), which refers to the food eaten on the grave of warriors, first recorded as the food eaten at the funeral of Atilla, who brought terror and a foreboding of extermination to the heart of Europe.

'Anxiety', on the other hand, overlaps with narrowness, constriction, constipation and a feeling of restricted space. 'Ankh', the Indo-European root of the word 'anxiety', meaning narrow and constricted, has a perfect counterpart in older languages. In ancient Egyptian, for example, the word for acute fear is composed of two symbols, one indicating narrowness and the other showing a man prostrate, as if dying. The latter symbol is also used to describe a severely wounded person. In Coptic, the meaning of constriction and narrowness conveys not only anxiety and mental pain, but also clinging and adhering. The words for fear and terror in these two languages connote immobility, helplessness, being chained while exposed to beating and punishment. The relationship to anguish and pain is obvious; the danger described by the concept of fear is expressed with greater force because it does not exist in the future but is very much part of the present.

In Arabic, the meanings of anxiety are similar to the Slavic. Various words are used – some referring to restlessness, others to constriction of chest or stomach. The synonym 'hasr', for example, when used as a noun, implies being besieged; but when used as a verb, denotes a state of being unveiled, without protection, without feathers so to speak – a state that requires hiding and avoidance of contact.

Other Arabic words for anxiety refer to somatic experience – 'ala' means difficulty in falling asleep or choking; 'lahvah' refers to problems with swallowing. However, none of these has a direct link to words for fear, which have a different set of synonyms describing states of trembling, jumping or being startled in response to something frightening.

Arabic and Slavic languages are also similar in the way in which they conceive extreme fear. In Arabic, terror contains the notion of immobility or of turning to stone. In Slavic 'strah' (fear) comes from the Baltic 'stregtt', meaning to turn to ice. Although climatic differences often contribute to variations in the symbolism, the images essentially describe the same behavioural response.

Images derived from the origins of words can best be traced in African and Far Eastern languages: in the former because they play a more important role than in European languages; in the latter (e.g. Chinese and Japanese) because pictographic writing is better equipped to preserve the origins of words. Etymological studies of Chinese characters have a long history and are enlightening, not only for the origins of signs in Chinese, but also for the study of the origins of words and concepts in general.

In Lingala, a language of the Bantu family spoken in Zaïre and the Congo, 'anxiety' is expressed as a wound in the heart, 'worry' as heaviness of heart, and 'terror' as the diminution or shrinking of a person with fear. In Chinese, the pictograph for anxiety and fear has several signs indicating an axe or cutting instrument and the heart. In Japanese, the word for anxiety is 'shimpai', a heart given away: however, the same word is also used for sorrow and for worry. All these perspectives of anxiety clearly describe feelings of unpleasantness, something that makes a person want to burst out, run away or start shouting or crying. To a degree, 'panic' overlaps this concept. The Japanese use the same symbol as the Chinese of a cutting instrument over a heart. 'Fear', on the other hand, is a separate concept and depicts breathlessness, and immobilisation of the vital force. In Fanti, a language spoken in Ghana, the word 'akomatu', which means 'panic', unites these images by defining a state in which the heart has flown away.

The elements of intensity and time are also viewed differently depending on the language. In Tagalog, a language spoken in the Philippines, 'fear' and 'terror' are differentiated by intensity, and both are differentiated from 'panic', which is distinguished by its rapid onset. 'Takot', the word for fear, is defined as a sense of danger. Terror, 'hilakbot', means extreme fear and panic and 'sindak' means sudden terror. 'Anxiety', or 'pagkabalisa' and 'pangamba', on the other hand, evokes uneasiness of mind and a premonition of danger. Other words related to anxiety, such as 'sabik' and 'pananabik', merely indicate impatience over delay – the elements of danger or fear are not evoked.

Conceptual equivalence

Conceptual equivalence is the second type of equivalence for consideration. It refers to the position and significance of the word in the theoretical system to which it belongs. 'Anger', for example, may be of great importance in one diagnostic system, but of marginal importance in another. Loss of face may be a reason for suicide in some cultures and irrelevant in others. Certain somatic or mental experiences are seen as a sign of disease in some cultures, while others pay little attention to them. Loss of semen, for example, is considered as an explanation for a variety of problems by patients in India. Koumare and colleagues (1992), when translating and testing a widely used self-report questionnaire, found that the item 'do your hands tremble' could not be used in a list of autonomic items in Mali because trembling of hands was considered as a sign of virility. 'Do you cry often?' was not usable because crying is a sign of weakness in a man, though not in a woman. Some of the items referring to somatic symptoms were difficult to interpret in a setting where many people suffer from diseases likely to cause similar symptoms. Other items, e.g. 'thought interference', seemed incomprehensible.

What is regarded as 'health' or 'illness' also varies across cultures and affects the meaning attached to experience and behaviour. Formulating an experience as part of an illness not only affects the behaviour of a patient, but also that of family members and others. It may influence the speed of referral and lead to difficulties in rehabilitation or to rejection of the patient. It may affect the willingness of people to discuss the problem, and the readiness of doctors to investigate its presence. Differences between the conceptual systems of health workers and patients can lead to misunderstandings and inappropriate management.

Thus composition of a questionnaire or of a semi-standardised instrument is determined by the authors' concepts of normality and disease in the population to be studied. Millennia of observation of morbid phenomena in a particular culture result in the definition of a universe of signs and experiences considered to indicate abnormality or illness in that context. Some of these signs and experiences, occurring together, are recognised as the symptoms of a named disease. Some of them are pathognomonic, i.e., their presence is sufficient to make the diagnosis. Others indicate abnormality in certain circumstances but not in others. Even when a phenonemon is seen as indicating abnormality or illness in both of two cultures that are being compared, the level of significance may vary.

Exploring conceptual equivalence can help to define what should be covered by an assessment instrument, and indicates ways in which the presence or absence of a phenomenon should be interpreted. Some information about conceptual equivalence can be obtained from anthropological investigation. It is also possible to gain relevant information from psychometric analyses. For example, a factor analysis of questionnaire data from Cattell's 16 PT test (1961) administered in English and French showed that the factorial structure remained the same when the test was used in French. However, some items 'changed' their place in the structure and 'belonged' to different factors in the two languages.

Technical equivalence

Technical equivalence is the third type of equivalence between two versions of a questionnaire. It refers to the way items should be used in order to obtain information. In England, for example, it is acceptable to ask a question such as 'What about your interests, have they changed at all?' The subject may answer by describing a loss of interest if this was indeed the case. In Uganda, Orley found it impossible to obtain more than a vague negative answer to this question; he had to change the form of enquiry to a dual exploration of a loss and an increase of interests (Orley and Wing, 1979). In Vietnamese and in some other languages there is no conditional tense; making it difficult to formulate questions illustrated by examples to clarify the interviewer's intent. In other cultures direct questioning about certain issues is not possible, and a circumspect manner of investigation is necessary.

Achieving technical equivalence is particularly difficult in the case of fully standardised instruments, which should theoretically be used in exactly the same manner by all interviewers. In semi-standardised interviews, in which the culturally appropriate meaning of an item is understood by the investigator, this difficulty can be avoided to a large extent. Clearly, the onus of ensuring cross-cultural technical comparability is then placed on training, so that investigators are clear as to the technical problems associated with each kind of rating.

Designing standardised and semi-standardised instruments with all three types of equivalence is even more complex when the instrument is to be used in more than two languages. The method most frequently used to achieve equivalence among three different language versions is to compare the two translated ones with the source version. If both are equivalent to the source, it is hoped that they will be equivalent between themselves. This is not necessarily the case. In a WHO study, the translations of a brief self-report questionnaire into several languages including Arabic, Spanish, English and Voloff were compared with the English original text. This was followed by an investigation of equivalence between the versions. The analyses showed that the different versions were, by and large, equivalent; there were however a few instances in which the source to target comparisons did reveal differences between the versions.

The most secure information about the level of equivalence of a clinical questionnaire or instrument in two languages can probably be obtained if bilingual clinicians interview bilingual patients. The design is not easy to use, and is even more difficult to apply if more than two languages are involved. Other methods of examining equivalence are less demanding and can give a fair estimate of comparability. These include the reiterative back-translation method, the committee method and the target check method, focus groups, interviews of key informants to obtain data about the meaning of words, and textual analyses in which the equivalence of a word is judged by whether it can be used in the same context in the two languages.

Combining the three types of equivalence

Over the years a combination of these methods has been applied to assess the equivalence of instruments used in WHO cross-cultural investigations. The blend of methods is different for semi-standardised instruments such as SCAN and for instruments with a completely standardised form of inquiry.

The first steps are similar for both. After the original version has been sufficiently well tested in the source language, it is submitted to a group of bilingual people, established for the purpose. The group should consist of experts skilled in interviewing and assessment, as well as clinicians and behavioural scientists, particularly anthropologists. The group will examine the overall form of the instrument and learn how to apply it. A skilled user of the instrument demonstrates its use and discusses its features with the bilingual group. Once the bilingual group has learned enough about the instrument to explain its nature and manner of application to other trainers, the bilingual experts meet with monolingual groups of future users and clinicians to discuss the translated version of the instrument. If no major problems are immediately visible to users and subjects, translation of the definitive instrument will be undertaken.

Monolingual groups are important because bilingual experts, who can guess the original meaning of the question, may well overlook practical difficulties in the form of the translated version. The monolingual groups should represent the range of likely interviewers and people with illness. Bilingual groups are important as 'committees' to discuss questions of semantic, conceptual and technical equivalence, for the translation of referred texts and as groups who can help with field testing to establish how the instrument is likely to perform.

Once the preliminary review has been completed, further work on the assessment of equivalence assumes different paths for the fully standardised and semi-standardised instruments. For the fully standardised instrument the next necessary step is a back-translation of the entire instrument into the original ('source') language. If there are differences, it may be necessary to amend the instrument, recheck its translation and carry out further back-translation, repeating the process until equivalence is achieved.

For semi-standardised instruments in which the main effort is directed at ensuring that the interviewers understand the nature of the items being rated and learn interviewing skills, it is sufficient to make target checks of carefully selected items. A list of items in the SCAN that should be included in the target check phase is given in Appendix 5.1. The list is not exhaustive, and should be expanded on the basis of results of reliability analyses and of discussions about the translation of SCAN into further languages (Sartorius, 1979).

The three stages of translation are summarised in Table 5.1.

Each of the components of SCAN requires separate exploration for instrumental equivalence. The clinical interview requires most attention. The Glossary helps interviewers to understand and remember the intended meaning of the items. The suggested probes have to be replaced, if necessary, by others with semantic, technical and conceptual equivalence.

Table 5.1 SCAN translation

Standardised	Semi-standardised and free

Creation of a bilingual group

↓

Familiarisation with the instrument.
Method of its application, etc.

↓

Establishment of monolingual
groups of users and subjects

↓

Translation

↓

Review by bilingual groups

↓

Review by monolingual groups
moderated by bilingual groups

↓

Discussion of monolingual findings
in bilingual groups

↓

Linguistic analyses

↓

First amendments in original text

↙   ↘

Full back-translation	Target check of items
↓	↓
Comparison of versions by central investigator	Target back-translation
↓	↓
	'Clinical' review
	↓
Iteration, if needed, with minor redrafts	Minor redrafts

↘   ↙

Review of translations with
redrafts by bilingual group

↓

Consideration of major changes:
Deletion or creation of new instrument parts

↓

Reliability and validity studies

↓

Final review by bilingual group

The rules for the formulation of these probes are fairly simple and include:

- Restrict each item to one topic of enquiry
- Use short sentences
- Use active rather than passive voice
- Use nouns rather than pronouns
- Avoid metaphors
- Avoid colloquial expressions used by subcultures
- Avoid conditional expressions
- Avoid the verbs could and would
- Avoid prepositions such as 'where' and 'when'
- Avoid possessive forms
- Avoid imprecise words such as 'probably'
- Avoid sentences with two verbs
- Avoid questions containing alternatives in the question

These suggestions supplement those for questions in survey instruments and they do not necessarily apply to the same degree for translations into all languages. Languages of the same family usually require less effort in achieving equivalence, although similarity in the form of a word often obscures dissimilarity of meaning.

Appendix 5.1   List of terms needing special attention when translating SCAN

activity

affect

age

amnesia

anxiety

anxious foreboding with auto-
    nomic accompaniments

associative states

attack

auditory hallucinations

autonomic anxiety

autonomic anxiety on meeting
    people

avoidance

black-out

borderline

brooding

changed perception of time
    including '*déja vu*'

choking

compulsive

concentration

conscious

consciousness

control

critical

delayed sleep
delusion
delusional confabulations
delusional memories
delusional mood
delusions of alien forces
    penetrating or controlling
    mind
delusions of assistance
delusions of catastrophe
depersonalisation
depressed mood
depression
derealisation
disability
disaster
disorientation
dissociative hallucinations
distortion
dizziness
doctor
drug-abuse
drug-dependence
dulled perception
early waking
elation
euphoria
exaltation
exhaustion
expansive mood
fantastic delusions
fatigue
foreboding
free-floating autonomic anxiety
fugue
grandiose ideas and actions
grimacing
guilty ideas of reference
hallucination
handicap

headache
heightened perception
high
hopelessness
hypersensitivity
hypochondriasis
ideas of reference
ideation
ideomotor pressure
impairment
incoherence
insight
intense
irreverent behaviour
irritability
keyed-up
lack of self-confidence with
    other people
loss of emotions
loss of interest
loss of libido
mannerism
marked
mild
moderate
moment
mood
morbid jealousy
morning depression
muscle pains
muscular tension
narrowing of repertoire
neglect due to brooding
nervous tension
obsessional checking
obsessional ideas and rumina-
    tion
pain
palpitations
panic

panic attacks
pathological guilt
perceptual distortion
perplexity
persecution
phobia
possession
posturing
poverty of content of speech
premenstrual exacerbation
reference
restlessness
self-confidence
self-conscious
self-depreciation
sensorium
simple ideas of reference
situational anxiety
social withdrawal

specific phobias
stereotypes
subjective anergia
subjective anergia and
    retardation
subjective ideomotor pressure
subjective feeling of nervous
    tension
subjectively inefficient thinking
suicidal plans
tension plans
thinking
thought echo
tiredness
trance
trembling
thought insertion
withdrawal
worry

References

Cattell R., Pichot P. and Rennes P. (1961) Constance interculturelle des facteurs de personnalité mesurée par le test 16 PF. Comparaison franco-américaine. *Revu Psychologie Appliquée*, 11: 165–96.
Kelly G. A. (1955) *A theory of personality*. New York: Norton and Co.
Koumare B., Diaoure R. and Miguel-Garcia E. (1992) Définition d'un instrument de dépistage des troubles psychiques. *Psychopathologie Africaine*, 24: 229–42.
Orley J., Wing J. K. (1979) Psychiatric disorders in two African villages. *Archives of General Psychiatry*, 36: 513–20.
Osgood C. E. (1952) The nature and measurement of meaning. *Psychology Bulletin*, 49: 197–237.
Pichot P. (1991) Personal communication.
Prince R. and Mombour W. (1967) A technique for improving linguistic equivalence in cross-cultural surveys. *The International Journal of Social Psychiatry*, 13: 229.
Sartorius N. (1979). Crosscultural Psychiatry. In: *Psychiatrie der Gegenwart*. Band I/1, 2. Heidelberg: Springer-Verlag.

Sartorius N. (1990) Cross-cultural and epidemiological perspectives on anxiety. In: Sartorius N. et al. *Anxiety–psychobiological and clinical perspectives*. Hemisphere Publishing Corporation.

Sartorius N. and Kuyken W. (1994) Translation of health status instruments. In: Orley J. and Kuyken W. (eds.) *Quality of life assessment: international perspectives*. Heidelberg: Springer-Verlag.

6   Technical procedures

T. B. Üstün and W. M. Compton III

Introduction

This chapter deals with the technical problems that must be solved in order to present for analysis the range of decisions made during the course of a clinical appraisal. The topics covered include the measurement of clinical course, the attribution of cause, the rating of interference with social function, the handling of multiple sources of information, the use of optional checklists, appendices and modules and the problem of missing data.

The basic principles are set out in the following text. The computer application discussed in Chapter 11 will provide more immediate on-line guidance.

'Periods' and 'episodes'

SCAN data are analysed on the basis of defined time periods within or across which episodes of disorder may occur. An *Episode* is a period of time throughout which clinically significant symptoms persist, with no symptom-free intervals lasting three months or more. It could last for a few days or for many years. SCAN provides two alternatives for rating time periods: a standard or routine option, and a free episode list. Dates are determined by clinical judgement. Each is described below.

The routine SCAN option

The routine option also provides a choice of two periods, one for the *present state* and one for *previous episodes*. Both periods can be rated in either PSE-10 or IGC.

In the current period only *Present State* (*PS*) can be rated.

For the previous period two options exist: *Representative episode*

(*RE*) and *Lifetime Before* (*LB*). The current period is rated in the left-hand box; *RE* or *LB* is rated in the right-hand box for each item.

Present State (PS)

When SCAN is used to structure the interview for a current period, the *Present State* (*PS*) represents a clinically significant disorder present during the month before the date of examination (approximately the last four weeks). As was the case with PSE-9, the term 'month' should be understood as notional or approximate; it could be extended up to 6 weeks or so, depending on the interviewer's clinical judgement. The episode need not have begun during the month; this would depend in part on the sample. The onset of *PS* could be years earlier. Therefore *PS* either constitutes an episode with an onset within the previous month, or is part of a longer episode. It can be used even when the disorder has persisted without a break for many years (even since adolescence), so long as the symptoms in *PS* are representative. The clinical picture in *PS* may be incomplete, as in residual depression or 'negative' schizophrenia. In that case *LB* is used as well.

The criteria for rating *PS* in persons with a current disorder are:

- that there should have been a clear period of 2 months without clinically significant symptoms immediately preceding the episode and no such period within it;
- clinically significant symptoms present within the notional month before interview.

The second of these criteria is important, since the disorder rated in the *PS* period should have enough clinically significant symptoms to provide a characteristic clinical profile and a diagnosis for the episode. Therefore, if the *Present State* is part of a continuous episode that has lasted longer than a month, with many characteristic symptoms still present but with a peak somewhat more than the 'notional month' ago, it is permissible to extend the period a little in order to accommodate the most characteristic symptoms within the *PS*. The most common occasion is likely to be when a patient has been admitted to hospital and has recovered to some extent before the interview. The number of days covered by the *PS* is always recorded.

When SCAN is used to structure the interview with people who do not have significant clinical symptoms at examination, the PSE should be completed for the previous month, consisting of all the above-cut-off items. This is called a *PS-check* and occurs most frequently:

- in a population or general practice survey, where many respondents will not be in episode as defined above:
- in clinical situations where acute episodes are infrequent, for example in follow up clinics, long-stay wards, day centres or hostels;
- when the disorder is only minor or takes the form of negative symptoms, and the most characteristic clinical symptoms have occurred in previous episodes.
- when long-term and clinically significant problems have lasted perhaps for years, but cannot be split up into episodes because fluctuations are not sufficiently marked. Examples might include very long-term dysthymic or somotoform disorders, and personality disorders with occasional minor symptoms. In such cases, the whole course of the condition constitutes one episode as defined in SCAN. Because significant symptoms are present during the month before examination, *PS* is the appropriate period to rate. If it lasts throughout the whole clinical course, from early adolescence, it is a form of 'lifetime ever'. However, it does not need a special designation since *PS* represents the whole course.

PS can be rated in the Item Group Checklist, from case-records or an informant, if the Respondent is unwilling or unable to supply information.

Previous Period

In *Previous Period*, any period of clinically significant symptoms could be rated. In order to separate it from the *Present State* any episode rated should occur with 2 or more months interval without significant symptoms before the *PS*, and similarly separated from any other episode by a clear 2+ month interval. However, in the case of bipolar disorder, periods of opposite polarity do not require the 2+ months interval. Two kinds of period are conventionally distinguished: *RE* and *LB*.

If there has been one particular episode before *PS* which, alone or in combination with *PS*, provides an adequate coverage of the significant clinical symptomatology for diagnostic purposes, it is dated and designated a *Representative Episode* (*RE*). *RE* will usually be used in association with *PS*. It can also be rated using the Item Group Checklist, if the Respondent is unable or unwilling to provide details and if good records and/or a good informant are available.

Three common uses for *RE* are:

- If the Respondent is in episode (*PS*) at the time of interview, and *RE* contains symptoms of similar type but with a more characteristic symptom profile, it will often be useful to rate both episodes: *PS+RE*.
- If *PE* and one particular *RE* contain different clinical pictures (for example, manic and depressive symptoms), the two sets of ratings will be processed separately, but the results of combining the two final outputs will also be reflected in the narrative printout.
- If R is not in episode at the time of interview (as confirmed by the *Check-PS*), *RE* is the chief source of information about a single past episode.

Lifetime Before (*LB*) is dated from the first onset of disorder to the beginning of the period covered in *PS*. *PS+LB* therefore constitute a form of 'lifetime ever'. *LB* is a period containing more than one episode and is mainly used in cases when there have been several previous episodes, whether discrete or merging into each other, that contain different types of symptom – e.g. psychotic, affective and neurotic – with the possibility of several diagnoses. It may then be necessary (depending on the nature of the *Present State*) to choose different peak periods for two or three episodes with different types of symptom but to rate them as though they were sub-episodes of one extended episode. The characteristic symptoms of each different type of previous episode are rated in one PSE-10 or IGC schedule, and each symptom type in *LB* is dated separately.

The routine CAPSE program processes the information as part of one episode, but, if sub-episodes are specified by symptom type and date, the relevant parts of the data can be identified for each separately. It should be emphasised that identifying the symptom type of an episode does not compromise the independence of the classification, since the CAPSE program does not take this information into account when categorising. It is, in any case, symptomatic, not diagnostic. Symptom scores and Item Group profiles, however, can only be provided for the whole of *LB*.

Full PSE-10 rating of more than 2 periods: the non-routine option

This option may be chosen instead of *PS/RE/LB*. Rating *LB* does not provide a full PSE profile for each type of disorder rated during the overall period. For projects that require this degree of detail, an 'episode list' should be completed instead of *PS* and *LB*.

This allows the specification of up to six dated episodes, each of which can be rated using the full PSE-10. Each episode is processed separately by CAPSE. It will not, however, be possible to link these episodes in a prose narrative as with the regular SCAN package. For some very detailed research projects, it may be useful to complete both the routine and the non-routine options for each member of the series.

Choosing the periods

Neurotic, affective and psychotic disorders

Sections of SCAN related to these disorders (subchapters F2–4 of ICD-10) are rated on the basis of one or two time periods, selected according to a flow chart. These rating periods represent episodes of disorder selected by the examiner (or pre-specified in a research project).

Other disorders

Most sections of SCAN are rated on the basis of one or two time periods, selected according to general principles that are described below. Four groups of conditions require a somewhat different procedure, which is fully specified in the text. These groups are:

Somatoform and dissociative disorders (Section 2)
The routine period for PS includes the past two years with provision for an earlier period.

Eating disorders (Section 9)
The routine period rated is the past year, but provision is also made for an optional earlier period to be specified by the examiner.

Alcohol (Section 11) and drug disorders (Section 12)
Two periods are specified – the year before interview and 'lifetime before'. Instructions are given in the interview text.

Cognitive disorders (Section 21)
Apart from a brief history section, these disorders are rated at examination.

The clinical history in SCAN

Methods of coverage

F0. Cognitive disorders

PSE-10 version 2, Section 21, is rated only for *PS*, with dates of onset and items for describing the course. Items in other relevant Sections are used to attribute causes.

F1. Alcohol and drug use disorders

PSE-10 Sections 11 and 12 are rated for the Past Year (*PY*) and/or Lifetime Before (*LB*), with dates of present and first onset. Items are included for attributing any F1 causation of symptoms rated elsewhere.

F20–42. Psychotic, affective and neurotic disorders

PSE-10 Sections 3–10, 16–19, 22–24 are rated for *PS*. A representative (previous) Episode (*RE*) OR Lifetime Before (*LB*) can also be rated, with dates of present and first onset. Special items are included for rating specific information needed to describe the course. PSE-10 Section 26 – the Item Group Checklist – can be used to rate such disorders from case records or informants.

F43–48. Stress, somatoform and dissociative disorders

PSE-10 Section 2 is rated for the past two years, with dates of present and first onset and specific course items.

F50. Eating disorders

PSE-10 Section 9 is rated for the Past Year (*PY*) and a previous episode, which can either be *RE*, if rated consistently throughout SCAN, or *LB* if rated over a different period to other previous episodes. Dates of present and first onset are needed.

F6–9

PSE-10 Section 27, the Clinical History Schedule, contains items for rating criteria needed for:

F6   Personality disorders
F7   Mental retardation and intellectual level

F8   Developmental disorders
F9   Disorders with onset in childhood
     Social roles and performance
     Social disablement

An independent clinical diagnosis, e.g. from case-records or another clinician, can also be recorded here.

Rating the course in SCAN

Onsets and durations

Dates and ages relating to various aspects of the course are entered in Sections 1 and 26. Throughout the SCAN text there are items for dating the onset of first episodes of specified symptom types. This topic is discussed further in chapter 10.

Specific rules concerning the course

Some ICD-10 and DSM-IV rules contain an instruction specifying certain time relationships between two or more symptoms or syndromes.

These rules are inserted as items in the relevant sections of SCAN text. Thus, item 6.030 deals with the number of depressive episodes; 6.031 with personality prior to the onset of depression; 6.032 with the severity of affective episodes; 6.033 with whether there have been two or more major depressive episodes followed by recovery, and 6.034 whether symptoms have shown a good response to adequate antidepressive therapy.

Rating these items does not affect the basic CAPSE classifications, only the relationships between them if present. All such items must therefore be rated if there is *any* likelihood that the disorders mentioned might be present.

The Item Group Checklist (Section 26) can be used when adequate information cannot be obtained from the respondent.

Use of the clinical history schedule is particularly useful in co-morbidity studies (i.e. categorical diagnosis or profile by childhood disorders, IQ, autism, sex, social status, occupation, disability, personality etc).

Attribution of cause in SCAN

Special and general guidance on the attribution of cause in SCAN version 2 is contained in Section 13 for Part One and Section 20 for Part Two, with an overall introduction on page 30. Instructions are given for attributions of physical, drug, substance and other organic causes, and for rating additional factors such as adolescence, migration, social deprivation etc. The Glossary elaborates these instructions.

An item level each SCAN item that may be caused by an exogenous factor is rated first for its severity. A separate rating may then be made of the etiological factor. In this way, ratings of phenomenology are separated from ratings of aetiology. At section level an attribution of cause is made at the end of each section of SCAN. The criteria used are as follows:

Organic cause of symptoms

If symptoms such as anxiety, obsessions, depression, hallucinations, delusions etc, are thought to be caused by organic factors, the attribution is made at the end of the relevant PSE-10 Section(s). Four criteria are applied:

- Evidence of cerebral disease, damage or dysfunction, whether direct or via non-cerebral disorder
- A presumed relationship between the development of disease and the onset of the mental disorder, such as onset within 3 months before or after the cerebral disorder
- Recovery or improvement after removal of the cause (a difficult criterion to meet)
- No other obvious cause

In most cases, there is one item for the attribution (Yes or No) and another to enter an ICD-10 code for the cause.

Attribution to psychoactive substance use

Attribution of substance-related cause is recorded with the ICD-10 code throughout SCAN-2.1.

Causes of overt cognitive disorders

The causes of disorders such as dementia, delirium, amnestic syndromes etc, are attributed in Section 21. Delirium due to alcohol or other psychoactive substance is attributed in Section 11 or 12 as well.

Additional factors influencing the manifestation of symptoms

These are listed, for Part One Sections, in Section 13 and, for Part Two Sections, in Section 20. They include:

Childbirth
Menopause
Bereavement
Adolescence
Special cultural group
Recent migration
Life events
Social deprivation

Interference with functioning

The degree to which symptoms in particular Sections interfere with everyday social and occupational functioning are mainly rated at the end of each section or in sections 13 and 20. An overall rating is entered at item 13.001 for Part One symptoms and at 20.048 for Part Two symptoms. A complete list is provided for Part One Sections at items 13.002–13.016. The most disabling symptom-type is chosen for entry.

Positive functioning

Provision is also made for rating positive functioning, as part of the procedure for determining cut-off points. This will be found most useful in community studies. It will also be useful, in co-morbidity studies, for examining the extent to which positive and negative ratings can coexist. Ratings for positive functioning can be made at items: 3.004 and 7.001.

Optional checklists, appendices and modules

Checklists are provided for certain conditions for which it is difficult to specify a detailed line of interviewing. The interview and examination are not standardised, but the items necessary for an ICD-10 and DSM-IV diagnosis are specified. The page numbers for checklists for stress and adjustment disorders, dysthymia and cyclothymia, brief depressive disorder, disorders associated with nondependency-producing drugs, schizotypal disorders, acute and induced psychoses, simple schizophrenia and mild cognitive disorder, are given in the list of contents. More detailed notes are provided in the Glossary.

Instruments associated with SCAN that can be used together with it or on their own are the International Personality Disorder Examination (IPDE) for ICD-10 and DSM-IV, sponsored by WHO. Modules concerned with sexual and gender disorders, cognitive disorders and neurological aspects of psychiatric disorders are in preparation.

Conventions used in SCAN

As in any instrument of the kind, numerous conventions are adopted to provide a standard format and make it reasonably easy to move around the documents once familiarity has been gained through repeated use. These are all fully explained in the various components of SCAN.

7 Training in the use of SCAN

T. B. Üstün, G. L. Harrison and S. Chatterji

SCAN trainers and training centres

Learning to use SCAN reliably requires a background of clinical experience followed by specialised training in a recognised training centre. An international network of centres has been developed to carry forward high-quality SCAN training in different languages and cultural settings. Just as SCAN itself is the culmination of a clinical tradition, flexible and adaptable to the needs of its users, SCAN training programmes allow a certain degree of flexibility to suit local needs and teaching styles. Nevertheless, to assure basic minimum standards and maintain quality control, training takes place within a basic organisational framework, and follows a core curriculum of specified skills and theoretical learning objectives.

Scan Training Centres are recognised because they have a minimum critical mass of staff experienced in the SCAN system and some track record of using SCAN in experimental field work. WHO Designated Training and Reference Centres must have adequate facilities for small group teaching, and facilities for demonstrating SCAN interviews with 'live' respondents and through video teaching materials. They also require well-organised administrative support to assist students where appropriate with accommodation and advice about local travel arrangements etc.

A *training manual* is available to SCAN trainers, setting the overall framework of teaching objectives, describing various teaching methods, and bringing together training materials and experience gained in different training centres. Although the manual outlines the range of core training objectives, it should be noted that the standardisation of training can be adaptable to the needs of local users.

It is recommended that SCAN trainers in WHO recognised training and reference centres should have had considerable experience of using the instrument, preferably in experimental field work, and normally they have participated in at least two courses at designated centres. Even experienced trainers should ideally participate in other courses from time to time to offer advice and feedback and to keep abreast of novel teaching methods and assessments. Trainers are normally prepared to participate in between-centre exercises co-ordinated by WHO, aimed at transcultural standardisation of the instrument, and other reporting procedures to allow the editorial committee to evaluate the progress of development of designated centres.

Training objectives

The object of SCAN training is to provide understanding of the definitions of symptoms and of how to acquire the ability to establish their presence or absence through clinical cross-examination. This complex task requires:

- A sound knowledge of basic psychopathology and a thorough knowledge of the Glossary definitions used in the SCAN system.
- experience and expertise in the application of the cross-questioning technique in establishing symptoms.
- the ability to make reliable judgements about the severity and duration of symptoms.

Because there are relatively complicated training requirements, SCAN training is 'objectives led' and based upon a curriculum. This is a plan fixing the goals of training and ordering the theoretical- and skills-based objectives within a logical framework. The SCAN curriculum summarises the irreducible minimum in terms of training aims; the central objectives aim to set standards for all trainees and for trainers.

Prerequisite level for SCAN trainees

Psychiatrists and psychologists with clinical experience who are familiar with different forms of psychopathology would be ideal candidates since they have skills in conducting clinical interviews. This is especially important for patients with psychotic symptoms who may pose particular challenges in understanding their experiences and carrying forward the detailed assessment in a way which is tolerable to the patient.

For Part One of SCAN, which deals with non-psychotic symptoms, non-clinicians who are educated in a mental-health related field (e.g. medical doctors or students, social workers, nurses) can also be reliable interviewers. Whatever their professional background however, potential SCAN trainees must be prepared to use and accept the Glossary definitions in SCAN and to follow the ground rules of clinical cross-examination. All SCAN students should also be willing to participate in group and individual supervision, and to have their ratings checked in order to maintain standardisation and reliability.

The SCAN curriculum

Although there will be some variation between SCAN training centres in terms of training methods, the objectives remain the same, and the curriculum (Appendices 7.1 and 7.2) outlines the central aims. It is based, first, on assessing what the student already knows and, second, on the acquisition of new clinical skills. The new learning will need to be consolidated during clinical practice subsequent to the training. It is recommended that students are provided with their own copy of the curriculum to enable them to pace their personal learning programme before and after the course.

SCAN training courses

The purpose of SCAN training is to enable trainees to reach the objective outlined in Appendix 7.1. In general two options have been adopted, although other types of course may eventually be adopted given the flexibility of the SCAN approach:

(a) *Short term (one week) courses*: these are generally condensed programmes in which groups of 4–12 people are trained by two trainers. This format is useful for those who need to travel to established institutions, and for larger research projects where groups of researchers can be trained together and reliability exercises planned and carried out.

(b) *Long-term courses*: these are weekly (or so) meetings that continue over 3 months or longer depending upon the number of sessions and hours per session. These are suitable for training resident trainees where there is a locally recognised training centre.

Conversion courses for previous PSE users have been suggested, since familiarisation with PSE-9 bears an advantage in grasping the basic features of SCAN. However, given the substantial revisions of PSE-10 and SCAN, the editorial committee have suggested that previous PSE-9 users should also participate in a standard scan training course.

A SCAN training course

A SCAN training course can be divided into 3 stages:

(a)   Pre-course preparations
(b)   The training course
(c)   Post-course activities

(a) Pre-course preparations

Preparation for the course is an important step in maximising the efficiency of the one week training period. Trainees should prepare themselves by reading the pre-course materials and learning the Glossary and basic features of the SCAN interview. The optimum use of the course depends upon adequate pre-course preparation both by teachers and trainees. Trainees should be provided with materials at least 4–6 weeks before the course, together with a trainee characterisation form to identify their background and research interests. This will enable the tailoring of the training programme according to the experience and needs of trainees. The information will normally include a brief curriculum vitae, experience of use of the PSE, familiarity with ICD-10 and DSM-IV and familiarity with computers. It will also be possible to request information about any specific research projects planned.

It would be advantageous to include the following in the pack of pre-course materials:

1   SCAN package including all components (PSE, IGC, GHS, Glossary, recording forms and output format).
2   SCAN computer assisted interview programmes (CAPSE) and its manual: a computer package which brings together the interview items, recommended probes, Glossary definitions and rating scales. The computer-assisted interview version may be useful in mastering the interview. It can be installed on a computer and may prove useful in tutorials because of its built-in functions such as immediate access to glossary and rating scales.

3 An introduction to SCAN, including written material and a video presentation outlining some of the main principles

4 SCAN Reference Manual: a comprehensive book which covers basic features of the SCAN system.

5 A copy of overheads which may be used during the SCAN training programme.

6 List of SCAN related publications demonstrating different uses of SCAN.

7 Description of the course including a timetable, instructions on how to prepare for the course (e.g. on what to read and how to approach the Glossary).

(b) The SCAN training course

Generally 8–12 trainees with at least two trainers are optimal for the 5-day course. This allows for most effective use of teaching time, space and training materials. Some centres have a pool of SCAN tutors, that is SCAN users with sufficient experience of the instrument to be able to supervise small-group learning with videos and live interviews. The basic aim of the course is the acquisition of the skill of constant reference to the Glossary and cross-examination of whether the subject's experience matches the pre-defined symptoms. Several methods and tools may be used:

A. Lectures

These are short introductory sessions given by experienced trainers, covering the basic structure of SCAN and its basic features. Trainers illustrate their material using overheads and video vignettes. In the early lectures trainees are orientated to the principles of 'structured' and 'standardised' interviews.

Overheads and other visual aids are especially useful in understanding the basic features of the SCAN system; for example, the utilisation of different periods may be illustrated by decision-making flow charts. These lectures are supported by books or handouts such as the SCAN instruction manual or other material on CIDI, IPDE, ICD-10 Checklist and ICD and DSM Classifications. Lectures are kept short and well focused, allowing plenty of time for interaction and focused discussion. The SCAN training manual has examples of case vignettes which may be used to stimulate discussion and to set homework assignments.

B. Demonstrations

Videotape recordings are particularly useful in showing the basic features of the interview and the principles of rating, since they can be stopped, replayed and discussed. A number of videotapes have been prepared as standard SCAN training materials and are contained in the SCAN training portfolio. This consists of a set of SCAN training materials which have been produced in WHO and in different training centres within the scan network. The training portfolio contains user instructions, exercises, overheads and lecture notes, together with a set of video presentations containing didactic material and illustrations from patient interviews.

The portfolio is accompanied by the SCAN training manual which sets out the terms of reference for SCAN training centres, guidelines on organising training courses and further instructions on using training materials.

C. Role-Playing

Practising interviews with improvised or written passages to learn the cross-questioning and rating styles is a useful introduction for trainees to begin using SCAN for themselves. Role-playing is best organised as a small group activity, preferably accompanied by a SCAN trainer or tutor. Practising interviews with one of the group members improvising a patient, or following set case vignettes allow trainees to be taught the principles of rating and to establish the importance of learning the Glossary thoroughly. Technical issues such as changes between rating scales and the question of attribution should also be discussed.

D. Observing live interviews with real subjects

Observing a skilled interviewer with a real respondent is an effective way to learn the basics of interviewing. It is better to place this exercise after the trainees have substantially grasped the basics of structured interviews. The trainees should rate this interview as observers and discuss agreement or disagreement on particular items.

E. Practical Work

The best way to learn SCAN is to use the instrument with a patient. Doing is learning. In attempting to use the instrument, trainees quickly establish the importance of knowing Glossary ratings, how to apply the schedules and how to solve problems. This should be attempted under the supervision of the trainer and only after trainees have undergone preliminary training, for example through lectures, observation of videos and trained interviewers and role-playing for themselves. In order to achieve better learning, ideally one should record ones own interviews and rate them critically with another member of the group or the supervisor. Feedback on interview techniques is very important: ideally the trainees should conduct interviews in pairs and discuss them with their peers and with SCAN trainers. If done thoroughly, such a discussion takes almost as long as the interview itself, so most training sessions should occupy some two hours.

The importance of learning the Glossary thoroughly must be repeatedly emphasised throughout the course. The Glossary delineates the signs and symptoms so that they can be recognised within the interview, identified and assessed. In order to have the item concepts formed in the mind of interviewers, there must be a basic overall review of the Glossary and constant reference to it during assessments.

Trainees naturally make a substantial number of errors during the learning period, and it should be stressed that we learn through making mistakes. The most common errors are pedanticity, misinterpretation of Glossary items and inadequate coverage of critical items. Inexperienced raters at first tend to rate a higher level of abnormality than experienced raters or trainers. The two other basic faults in rating are the halo effect (rating the associated symptoms as positive) or the carry-over effect (drawing premature conclusions about the presence or absence of a diagnostic syndrome and rating other symptoms accordingly). The only way to correct these errors is by way of observation, warning and critical discussion. Details are given in Chapters 5 and 6.

F. Group Learning
Generally SCAN training takes place in small groups. Mechanisms of group learning and team work are an important means of training. In a group, trainers talk to students, talk *with* students, have them talk *together*, show students *how*, supervise them and provide opportunities for practice. This not only keeps the motivation of the trainees (and trainers) high, but also provides a rich media for feedback. Feedback to the learner is important, because in this way the trainees

acquire the common norms for rating which form the basis of standardisation. In this context, it is useful to make a consensus rating session at the end of an interview where group ratings generally represent standard ratings.

A sample timetable which has been developed by WHO following consultation with experienced SCAN trainers is given in Appendix 7.3. This should be taken as a flexible schedule, and the order of activities tailored to the needs and previous experience of the trainees, and teaching styles of trainers.

SCAN trainers should utilise active group teaching methods (e.g. role-playing) as much as possible to teach basic principles of interviewing, and illustrate common pitfalls. The course time should be devoted to practice sessions and live interviews to the maximum extent possible.

Some practical aspects of organising a course

Trainers who organise courses for teaching SCAN should have the following items prepared for use during the course:

(a) Live respondents to demonstrate full SCAN interviews. Live interviews are the main stay of SCAN training.

(b) Video recordings illustrating all SCAN sections: since it may be difficult to find different patients to demonstrate all components of the SCAN examination systematically, videos should be prepared which can be used in full or in part. Video clips which bring together different examples to some items can enrich the repertoire of trainees and assist in making comparative ratings. Furthermore, each trainee should rate 'master' tapes that are already rated by experienced interviewers and selected for training purposes. Ratings can then be compared with experts' consensus ratings.

(c) Computer programs: diagnostic programs (CATEGO-5 and algorithms, computer assisted interview).

(d) Sample SCAN outputs and annotated examples.

(e) ICD-10 and DSM-IV handbooks.

(f) Training exercises (homework).
It is recognised that 'details' of organisation can make an important contribution to the success or otherwise of a course. Students should have clear directions, regular breaks for refreshments and should not be kept 'waiting around' for patients due to poor organisation.

Quality control in SCAN training

Quality control of training is given a high priority within the SCAN training network.

A Multiple Choice Questionnaire (MCQ) based on Glossary definitions may be a useful local instrument on the first day of the course. The aim of the MCQ assessment is to emphasise the importance of pre-course preparation by giving prior notice of this relatively short and simple test of grasp of some basic Glossary definitions. The MCQ format will allow rapid marking so that results can be returned to students early in the course, allowing a general discussion about queries that have arisen and any weaknesses revealed in their scores.

The student evaluation and feedback schedule evaluates the effectiveness of SCAN training in terms of its impact on students' perceived self-efficacy. Self-efficacy refers to individual expectations of mastery or competance to perform specific behaviours (e.g. interview skills) needed to influence desirable outcomes (e.g. accurate diagnosis). With respect to SCAN training, it will be valuable to know whether students show increased self-efficacy for diagnostic interviewing following the SCAN training experience, and, by collecting data from large numbers of trainees over time, it will become possible to identify training modules, exercises and training procedures that are optimal for improving trainees' competence.

Trainers are encouraged to conduct a formal review of each course to identify strengths and weaknesses in their training materials and methods.

Certification or qualification

WHO-designated SCAN training in reference centres provides evidence of attendance at the course, but certification is a problematic issue. The scientific way to assess effective learning is to establish reliability between two interviewers: it is not only difficult to assess reliability during a short training course, but such an attempt may itself block the learning process. Researchers should provide the evidence of acceptable interreater reliability only after they have fully mastered the interview. Such an exercise would be better carried out after the training course, and preferably in the research setting itself. The SCAN training certification therefore certifies attendance at a course, but does not offer any judgement about the expertise or otherwise of any individual trainee. In assessing any paper which gives results based on the use of SCAN, the reader should always take into account the training of the interviewers and the evidence for reliability. Intercentre reliability requires separate protocols.

After-course activities

(1) It should be noted that the course itself is not of sufficient length to master the full SCAN, and interviewers should be called upon to carry out a minimum of twenty interviews so as to optimise their experience. Quite a large proportion of learning in the SCAN course itself goes into familiarisation with the schedule contents and order of questions. Only then does it become possible to keep closely to the schedule (which literally must be known by heart) while still maintaining a natural and easy manner of questioning, sympathetic comments and additional minor probes.

(2) Interviewers should then rate a certain number of audiotapes and videotapes for reliability assessment. In order to establish a sufficient degree of reliability, a set of test tapes are included in the SCAN training portfolio. These 'master' tapes may then be rated by experienced interviewers, and selected for training purposes together with consensus ratings.

(3) Use of computer programs requires hands-on experience. The training course gives an introduction to the use of the computer programs, and some trainees may prefer to use them throughout the course rather than learn in hard copy. Clearly, however, consolidation will be necessary after the course.

(4) Participation in post-course follow-up meetings (booster sessions) is an ideal method of consolidation. Some training and reference centres offer follow-up meetings within annual national congresses, where trainees meet for technical discussions and booster sessions after having completed their personal training.

(5) WHO has established a web site on diagnostic instruments which announces research projects and training calendars, and gives an updated list of SCAN-related publications (www.who.ch\scan).

(6) Establishment and use of SCAN databanks: WHO has established a data library where SCAN and CIDI data are brought together from different studies together with study descriptors. This allows, within certain limits, comparisons of psychopathology at item level.

(7) A problem hotline and problem reporting sheet: some SCAN training and reference centres are able to provide a problem hotline where trainees can call or fax their query about an interview and the computer programs. A standard form has been developed for reporting problems to provide feedback for the development of the instrument, the manuals and computer programs.

The training courses and training materials are organised by WHO designated SCAN training and reference centres, and there is a special editorial committee to overlook the training needs and standardisation issues as well as future developments in SCAN.

Appendix 7.1   The SCAN training curriculum

PART A. Theoretical learning objectives

(1) At the end of SCAN training students should *understand*:

- the meaning of standardised and semi-standardised interviews

  - the use of standardised instruments in clinical and epidemiological research

- the basic outline of other standardised and semi-standardised instruments including CIDI and IPDE
- the development of the PSE (including PSE-10) and its use in major research projects
- the central components of PSE-10 as a standardised instrument

  - bottom-up approach
  - although substantially structured retains the features of a clinical examination
  - Glossary at the heart of the SCAN requirement for standard definitions
  - the rules governing clinical cross-examination

- the rules for rating severity
- the options and rationale for rating different periods

- issues in cross-cultural assessment

  - the scope and limitations of the translation procedures used with SCAN
  - problems of Glossary definitions in different cultural setting

- the two main diagnostic systems linked to SCAN: ICD-10 and DSM-IV

  - the rationale for operational research criteria
  - similarities and differences between the systems
  - outline knowledge of the meaning of algorithms and their application to developing diagnoses within the SCAN system

(2) At the end of SCAN training students should have a *working knowledge of*:

- the definition of each SCAN item as given in the Glossary
- the 3 main episodes rated in SCAN – their meaning and application
- the 4 rating scales used in SCAN – the student must understand the reason for their complex structure and the requirement for special rating on some items
- the purpose of the special episode rating
- the overall structure of SCAN: Parts One and Two, and the function of cut-offs
- numbering and naming of the 27 sections in SCAN
- the optional ratings for aetiological attribution etc.
- nature and purpose of the Item Group Checklist (IGC) recording information from collateral sources
- nature and purpose of the Clinical History Schedule (CHS). The options (including their limitations) for recording estimates of childhood and other developmental disorders, level of intellectual functioning, social function and confidence ratings.
- the CATEGO computer scoring program for SCAN used to generate ICD-10 and DSM-IV diagnoses, provisions for descriptive scores and profiles, the algorithms for 'caseness' and diagnostic classification
- different formats for recording ratings
- the use of the CAPSE programs and manuals (see Chapters 9 and 11) for conducting interviews and recording data

PART B. Skills learning objectives

(1)   At the end of a SCAN training, students should have acquired a *basic level of skill* in examining a patient respondent. They should demonstrate basic skills in:

- using the SCAN manual (or the CAPSE program if applicable) whilst interviewing; following cut-offs and moving reasonably quickly between sections;
- eliciting symptoms through the process of clinical cross-examination with a patient respondent; matching the Glossary definition of symptoms to the experience of the patient and making appropriate ratings for presence or absence of symptoms;
- applying the ground rules of PSE clinical examination with a patient respondent:
  - using opening probes, followed by flexible use of suggested probes
  - recording examples of symptoms
  - when in doubt, rate down;
- Choosing appropriate periods for ratings;
- controlling the patient in order to progress the interview whilst supporting the patient and showing understanding of his/her distress;
- making ratings in at least one of the recording formats and entering data into the CATEGO program; understanding the output and reference classifications.

Appendix 7.2   Sample overview for SCAN training course

I   **Introduction to Principles of Diagnosis, classification and interviewing**
2 hrs

II   **Introduction to SCAN** – including historical evolution and development, current status, principles, organisation, philosophy, components and options.
2 hrs

III **Discussion of the SCAN Glossary** – including principles, comparison to other descriptions and review of items of special importance.
4 hrs

IV   **Review of the SCAN interview section by section** – using overheads,

role-plays, video interviews, ratings, demonstration of live subjects
and home exercises.

15 hrs

V   **Live interviews by participants** – including actual supervised interviews of subjects in small groups by trainees, rating and discussion.

16 hrs

VI   **Introduction to computer applications** – including demonstration of CAPSE and CATEGO-5.

1 hr

VII   **Issues in translation and adaptation**

1 hr

VIII   **Introduction to other interview schedules** – IPDE/CIDI
IX   **Brief review of ICD-10/DSM-III-R/DSM-IV**

1 hr

Appendix 7.3   Sample training programme

Day 1

Morning
Welcome and introduction, followed by:

Lecture: Introduction to SCAN:

a.   purposes, principles, components of SCAN
b.   recording forms and outputs
c.   course ratings
d.   selection of episodes; date of onset; special items in IGC and CHS; organic causes; precipitants, checklists, stress disorders; limitation on activities
e.   explain architecture of Sections 1, 13, 14 and CHS (overheads)

Video 1:

a.   interactive display
b.   discussion of Video 1 (overheads)

Afternoon
Introduction to Glossary:
a.   clinical interviewing using Glossary definitions

b. principles of cross-examination
c. examination of Glossary definitions
d. core and principles of Glossary: reference points

Day 2

Morning

Mini-lecture: Structure of ICD-10 classification

Live interview: Clinical interview using SCAN (A case of simple depression – first episode)

a. explain architecture of sections 3–8 (overheads)
b. display Video 1 uninterrupted
c. discussion: interactive replay of Section 3 from Video 1 with overheads.
    Concentrate of interview techniques, rules and Glossary definitions
d. rating scale I: recording ratings
                  explain 4 fixed formats
                  (Interview booklet,
                  Coding Booklet, named
                  Coding Booklet, unnamed
                  Free format Coding
                  Computer Assisted Interview Coding)
e. interactive rerun Video 1: rating items
f. outputs of Video 1 (overheads).

Afternoon

Interview/Video 2: Anxiety Section: panic

a. explain architecture of Section 4 and (2–5) (overheads)
b. display Video 2 uninterrupted
c. discussion of Video 2: (overheads) interview techniques, ratings, outputs

Exercises: Using Rating Scale I: Rating sections 6, 7, 8.

Day 3

Morning

Lecture: Structure of DSM-IV Classification; Introduction to Section 2

Interview/Video 3: Physical health and somatoform disorders

a. explain architecture of Section 2 and key items (overheads)
b. display Video 3 uninterrupted
c. discussion of Video 3: (overheads) interview techniques, ratings, outputs

Introduction to Section 5

Interview/Video 4: Obsessions

a. explain architecture of Section 5 (overheads)
b. display Video 4 uninterrupted
c. discussion of Video 4: (overheads) interview techniques, ratings, outputs

Afternoon
Introduction to Section 10

Interview/Video 4: Mania

a. explain architecture of Section 10 (overheads)
b. display Video 4 uninterrupted
c. discussion of Video 4: (overheads) interview techniques, ratings, outputs

Review progress with the group.

Exercises: Rating exercises on Sections 2, 3, 4, 5.

Day 4

Morning
Lecture: CIDI (Composite International Diagnostic Interview)

Interview/Video 5: Psychoactive substance abuse (Alcohol)

a. explain architecture of Sections 11 and 12 (overheads)
b. display Video 5 uninterrupted
c. discussion of Video 5: (overheads) interview techniques, ratings, outputs

Interview/Video 5: Psychoactive substance abuse (Drugs)

a. explain architecture of Sections 11 and 12 (overheads)
b. display Video 5 uninterrupted
c. discussion of Video 5: (overheads) interview techniques, ratings, outputs

Afternoon
Interview/Video 5: SCAN Part One Overview: full interview

Present State and Representative Episode
A Bipolar Case (s 6–10) or depression with anxiety (s 2–5)

a. recapitulation of SCAN Part One (overheads)
b. discussion (overheads) rules for period selection interview techniques, ratings CHS, completing Part One

Interview/Video 6: Psychotic Sections (Part Two)

a. explain architecture of Sections 16 to 19 (overheads)
b. display Video 6 uninterrupted
c. discussion of Video 6: (overheads) interview techniques, ratings, outputs

Introduction to behavioural items

Video 7: Behavioural items: a pot-pourri

a. explain architecture of Section 16 to 19 (overheads)
b. display Video 7
c. discussion of Video 7: (overheads) definitions, ratings

Exercises: Rating exercises on Sections 1, 10, 11, 12, 13, 14.

Day 5

Morning
Lecture: IPDE (International Personality Disorder Examination)

Video 8: SCAN Parts One and Two: full interview

Present State and Lifetime Before
A psychotic case with negative symptoms and previous florid symptoms

a. explain architecture of episodes (overheads)
b. display Video 8 uninterrupted
c. discussion of Video 8: (overheads) interview techniques, ratings of CHS, completing Parts One and Two

Video 9: Cognitive assessment in SCAN

A case of mild dementia

a. explain architecture of Section 20 (overheads)
b. display Video 9 uninterrupted
c. discussion of Video 9: (overheads) interviews techniques, ratings, outputs

Afternoon
Review of computer programs:

a. data entry
b. diagnostic programs: ICD, DSM, and CATEGO-5
c. outputs

Life after the SCAN course:

a. how to keep in touch
b. SCAN network

Exercise: Rating exercise on Part Two: Sections 15–24.

8 International field trials: SCAN-0

J. K. Wing, N. Sartorius, G. Der and participating Field Trial Centres

Reliability of earlier editions of the PSE

Earlier version of the PSE have been extensively tested in a wide range of working conditions. An early scepticism, reasonably based on studies showing that free clinical interviews did not produce comparable diagnostic results from different examiners interviewing the same series of patients (Kreitman, 1961; Zubin, 1967), was dispelled by data using PSE-3-PSE-5 (Wing et al., 1967), which demonstrated high concordance between interviewer–observer pairs and between different interviewers examining the same patient. Kendell and colleagues (1968) using PSE-7 confirmed these results. The same scepticism had to be overcome when choosing an instrument for the USA–UK Diagnostic Project and the International Pilot Study of Schizophrenia. PSE-7 and PSE-8 were successfully and reliably used in both projects (Cooper et al., 1972; WHO, 1973; Wing et al., 1974). The experience did demonstrate, however, the need for more precise definitions and instructions when examiners from a wide range of backgrounds were collaborating in an international study. Luria and colleagues (1974, 1979) also demonstrated that the system could be used reliably in the United States.

PSE-9 has been further tested in numerous projects throughout the world. Reliability of scores and classifications has been found to be good in a wide range of conditions, including general population samples and most types of clinical setting (Bebbington et al., 1981; Cooper et al., 1977; McGuffin et al., 1986; Pakaslahti, 1987; Rogers and Mann, 1986; Sturt et al., 1981; Wing et al., 1977; Wing et al., 1978). A full discussion of the concept of reliability as it affected the PSE-9 used in a follow-up of the IPSS series has been provided by Gulbinat (1979).

The prototype for SCAN

The Chart in Chapter 2 shows the progression of SCAN through four consecutive versions: 0, 1, 2.0 and 2.1. The first working draft of a prototype (not then named) was dated September 1983. It incorporated most of the changes in design described in Chapter 2, and was adopted following pilot interviews with short-term and long-term patients in a variety of hospital and community settings. This prototype was used in a study of the needs for care and services of 145 people attending day hospitals and day centres for more than a year, living in a deprived area of south-east London, aged 18 and over, and not suffering from dementia or severe mental retardation (Brewin and Wing, 1988; Brewin et al., 1987, 1988; Brugha et al., 1988). The study provided a severe test of the ability of the new instrument to take the clinical history into account, since attenders had been in contact with services for an average of 15 years, and nearly half did not have conditions that could be diagnosed from a Present State interview alone.

Some results from this study are relevant to the subsequent development and interpretation of SCAN results. The prototype CATEGO-5 was modified from CATEGO-4 for ICD-8 diagnoses (ICD-9 was closely similar), since ICD-10 categories had not then been specified. One set was derived from the 'present state' (a draft version of PSE-10 for the past month) and another from an earlier representative episode (RE) or 'lifetime before' (LB) using drafts of the Item Group Checklist and Clinical History Schedules. There was a good (89%) concordance between three groups of SCAN and independent hospital diagnoses—psychotic, affective and neurotic (N 108). However, in the other 37 cases (26% of the 145) one or other diagnosis was of personality disorder, brain syndromes, mental retardation, autism, or unclassified, most not derivable from SCAN.

The problem of the classification of chronic disorders is discussed in Chapter 1. This series made clear the importance of the dimensional approach made possible by the range of Item Group and Symptom Type (ST) scores, which provide a complementary and comprehensive description of the Present State. The results of a principal components analysis of 12 ST scores are shown in Table 8.1. The scree test (Cattell, 1966) indicated four factors, with eigenvalues of 3.26, 2.52, 1.53 and 1.25, accounting for 71% of the variance. They are readily identified: 1, Depression and Anxiety; 2, Schizophrenia

Table 8.1. *Principal components analysis of Prototype symptom scores for Present State. Patients attending long-term day care. N 145*

| Present State ST scores | Factors and loadings | | | |
	1 DA	2 SP	3 MN	4 NG
Schizophrenic delusions and hallucinations		0.87		
Other delusions and hallucinations		0.80	0.37	
Mania and hypomania			0.71	−0.38
Depressed mood	0.92			
Anxiety and phobias	0.67	−0.22		
Nonspecific neurotic symptoms	0.91			
Negative signs				0.82
Other speech disorder			0.73	0.44
Other behaviour disorder		0.24	0.82	0.23
Other affective disorder		0.42		0.51
Other perceptual disorder	0.46	0.64		
Subjectively experienced slowness	0.84			

Notes:

DA Depression and Anxiety   SP Schizophrenia and Paranoid
                                        Psychosis
MN Mania   NG Negative signs

Factor loadings with absolute values <0.20 omitted

and Paranoid Psychoses; 3, Mania; 4, Negative Signs. There were only 4 cases of mania, but all were acute and typical. The loadings clearly differentiated subjectively experienced slowness (factor 1) from negative signs in behaviour (factor 4). Positive symptoms of schizophrenia in the Present State did not have a loading on factor 4 in this long-term population.

Table 8.2 shows the relationship between overall prototype diagnoses (taking history into account) and factor scores based on the present clinical state. A classification as schizophrenia (often based on positive symptoms experienced years earlier) had a high score on factor 4 (negative signs). So also did class 9 (other disorders; including mild mental retardation and Asperger's syndrome),

Table 8.2. *Mean factor scores for Prototype overall diagnostic classes*
Patients attending long-term day care. N 145

Overall classification	No. LE	No. PS	Factor scores (PS)			
			1 DA	2 SP	3 MN	4 NG
Schizophrenia	52	21	−0.16	0.60	−0.09	0.30
Paranoid psychosis	18	15	−0.46	−0.02	−0.15	−0.06
Retarded depression	14	12	0.98	−0.25	−0.28	−0.24
Mania and bipolar	21	4	−0.07	−0.32	0.58	−0.47
Other depression	9	8	1.10	−0.39	−0.33	−0.43
Anxiety and phobia	6	13	0.73	−0.75	−0.08	−0.67
Personality disorder	6	25	−0.22	−0.34	0.23	−0.19
Unclassified	9	46	−0.33	−0.46	−0.20	0.23
Other disorder	10	1	−0.58	−0.63	0.27	0.63
Total	145					
Significance (Anova)			<0.001	<0.001	0.183	0.011

Notes:
The scores are based on Present State items but calculated for the overall diagnoses

PS Number in category based on Present State
LE Number in category based on PS + previous history

while the affective and anxiety disorders had scores well below the mean.

Further analysis showed that a rating of long-term social disablement, equivalent to the term 'handicap' in the IDH classification (WHO, 1980), made from case-records, was highly associated with an overall SCAN diagnosis of schizophrenia and with the score representing negative signs in the Present State.

The components of SCAN version 0 used in the field trials (February 1988) were developed from the prototype bearing these results in mind, together with comments and suggestions from a broad and international range of clinicians consulted by the WHO/ADAMHA Task Force on Diagnostic Instruments (see Chapter 2).

WHO field trials of SCAN-0

Field trials of SCAN-0 were undertaken under the auspices of WHO, after key participants from 17 centres, in 14 countries, had been trained to use the third (February 1988) draft. The English text was translated into 10 other languages, based on the principle that it was more important to translate the concepts than the words (see Chapter 5). Independent back-translation of the key items was used as a check.

The training and co-ordinating Centre was the MRC Social Psychiatry Unit at the Institute of Psychiatry in London.
The following Centres took part:

Ankara	Geneva	Mannheim
Athens	Groningen	Nottingham
Bangalore	Leicester	Santander
Beijing	London	Sofia
Canberra	Lübeck	Sao Paolo
Farmington		Sydney

Early results of the trials were reported at the World Congress of Psychiatry in 1990 and published in the proceedings.

Extra trials were undertaken of the eating, substance use and cognitive sections, which were not sufficiently tested in the main series because of lack of numbers or substantial changes in the SCAN-0 text:

Cognitive disorders:	Athens, Santander
Alcohol and drug use:	Århus, Ankara, Sofia, New York
Obsessional disorders:	Sydney

Design of the trials

The design of the trials was agreed at the first two training meetings in London in November 1987 and March 1988. Each centre would collect 20 consecutive or representative patients admitted to hospital or seen at the start of some other episode of contact with specialist services. They would also, according to agreement, collect a further 10 with some particular clinical pattern of symptoms. F0 disorders were excluded, since the relevant section had not been finalised in time. At least three interviewers would take part, taking it in turns to conduct the examination. At the first examination, there would always be an interviewer and independent observer rating the present state (Pair 1). The same two participants would also rate a second period if necessary (Pair 2). A follow-up interview would be conducted within two weeks for 20 patients, the examiner not being the same as on the first occasion (Pair 3, different interviewers on the two occasions). It was assumed that a previous period, if used, would often be rated with the Item Group Checklist (Pair 4). A wide range of types and severity of disorder was expected given these conditions.

Table 8.3 shows the numbers of respondents and rater pairs by Centre. The total number of people interviewed using PSE-10 was 478. All Centres but two produced 20 or more pairs of initial interviewer–observer schedules for analysis. Fewer than expected (N 125, 25%) completed a schedule for an earlier period; the information available in the present state being sufficient for a diagnosis. A follow-up was achieved in 236 cases (Pair 3, 49%). The IG Checklist was used by a pair of interviewers in only 28 cases; insufficient for analysis.

The age distribution was as follows:

<20, 8%; 21–40, 56%; 41–60, 29%; 61+, 7%.

Age distribution was roughly similar between Centres except that there were more in the 41–60 category in Canberra, Leicester, Nottingham and Sydney, where fewer people with schizophrenia were included. There were 49% men and 51% women.

Feasibility and acceptability

Feasibility and acceptability were judged to be good, though the interview could be substantially longer than PSE-9 because of the extra coverage and the option for rating more than one period. On average, the interviewer took an hour and a quarter, much depending on whether one period or two was rated and whether the alcohol and drug sections needed to be used. A maximum of 2h 30m was recorded. Problems were also experienced with items governing the rules for the type of course the disorders were following, particularly for DSM-III-R items. The layout of the section on anxiety symptoms was found to be too complicated, which probably detracted from reliability. Many detailed comments were made on the substance use and cognitive sections, and a general complaint was filed about the lack

Table 8.3. *SCAN-0: Field Trial Centres*
Numbers of respondents and rater pairs

Centre	N resp.	N Pair 1 PSE	N Pair 2 PSE	N Pair 3 PSE	N Pair 4 IGC
Ankara	30	30	9	20	6
Athens	30	30	4	24	13
Bangalore	30	30	1	–	–
Beijing	20	–	–	–	–
Canberra	30	30	5	15	1
Farmington	24	24	24	17	–
Geneva	32	31	7	22	–
Groningen	30	30	–	25	–
Leicester	30	30	–	25	–
London[a]	33	27	1	15	–
Lübeck	19	10	–	4	–
Mannheim	26	26	–	–	–
Nottingham	30	30	3	9	–
Santander	30	30	26	20	4
Sao Paolo	31	29	12	20	4
Sofia 20	20	–	20	–	–
Sydney	33	33	33	–	–
Total	478	440	125	236	28

Notes:

[a] Seven London cases used in demonstrations are omitted

Pair 1: Interviewer and Observer, Period 1, PSE
Pair 2: Interviewer and Observer, Period 2, PSE
Pair 3: Interview (Period 1) and Interviewer (Follow up), PSE
Pair 4: Two raters using Item Group Checklist

of a detailed section on somatoform and dissociative symptoms. Much subsequent development work was based on these comments.

ICD-10 and DSM-III-R

Diagnoses from the two systems were obtained by applying CATEGO-5 to the same set of SCAN data. Table 8.4 shows the numbers of ICD-

Table 8.4. *SCAN-0: ICD-10 and DSM-III-R classification*

ICD-10 code	Diagnostic group and mnemonic[a]		N ICD-10	N DSM-III-R
F20.0–4	SZ	Schizophrenia	103	76
F25	SZAF	Schizoaffective	1	5
F22	DL	Delusional psychosis	25	23
F30–31	MNBP	Mania and bipolar	44	51
F32–34	DP	Depressive disorders	153	131
F40	PB	Phobias	12	29
F41	PNGA	Panic and anxiety	13	14
F42	OB	Obsessional disorder	3	7
F50.0	ANEX	Anorexia nervosa	8	6
F50.1	BLIM	Bulimia nervosa	4	2
F10.1	HMAL	Harmful use of alcohol	62	63
F10.2	DDAL	Dependence on alcohol	6	6
F1x.1	HMDG	Harmful use of drug	21	19
F1x.2	DDDG	Dependence on drug	4	4

Notes:
Diagnoses in the bottom part of the table can co-exist with those in the top part
[a] These mnemonics are also used in subsequent tables

10 and DSM-III-R diagnoses derived from the Pair 1 interviewer's PSE-10 ratings (present state). It demonstrates the expected lower number of cases of DSM-III-R schizophrenia and higher numbers of bipolar disorder.

Reliability of SCAN-0 in field trials

Overall concordance on the set of items needed for a particular diagnosis can be assessed by calculating the degree of agreement between two sets of ratings of the same interview or the same patient interviewed twice. Factors influencing the reliability of rating SCAN items include:

a. variation in a patient's state over time;
b. variation in reporting: the patient may give different information to different examiners;
c. examiner variation: different information may be obtained by different styles of examination;
d. observer variation: raters may vary in their understanding or interpretation of the phenomena.

The first two are not sources of examiner error, but do contribute to the design of the reliability test. The other two can be limited by training.

Apart from the conventional kappa, a purely descriptive index is used to express degree of agreement. This is the positive Index of Association (IA$_p$) or Chamberlain's p_{pos}, 'an index of proportionate positive agreement' (Cicchetti and Feinstein, 1990; Maxwell, 1977; Wing et al., 1977). It is calculated as the number of cases in which the two sets of data yield the same category expressed as a percentage of the total number so categorised. The number not categorised from either data-set is omitted in the tables, but a negative index based on the absence of the category, calculated in equivalent fashion, would usually be higher.

Concordance between ICD-10 categories

Table 8.5 shows the results of applying the CATEGO-5 program for ICD-10 to data-sets derived from three pairs of raters. Pair 1 and Pair 2 were usually the same for each patient for whom two periods were rated, but sometimes the examiner and observer changed roles. The examiner in Pair 3 was always different to the examiner in Pair 1. Only categories containing 10 or more cases were considered.

For Pair 1, the kappa coefficients for ICD-10 diagnoses are above 0.60. Hazardous drinking and drugtaking were subsequently removed from ICD-10 and are not included in the tables. Anxiety disorders (kappa = 0.60) should be more reliably rated in the revised format. The kappa for delusional psychosis is 0.63, due to overlap with other psychoses and affective disorders. Analysis of dis-

Table 8.5. *Agreement between Pairs on CATEGO-5 ICD-10 classes*

Diagnostic group[a]	Pair 1			Pair 2			Pair 3		
	N^b	$IA_p{}^c$	Kappa	N	IA_p	K	N	IA_p	K
SZ	101	89	0.93	13	77	0.86	46	63	0.73
SZAF	[d]1								
DL	25	48	0.63	[d]8			18	17	0.25
MNBP	48	73	0.83	15	57	0.92	36	51	0.62
DP	154	86	0.89	33	88	0.91	111	70	0.71
PB	16	69	0.81	[d]9			[d]2		
PNGA	18	42	0.60	[d]6			10	20	0.32
OB	[d]4								
ANEX	10	70	0.82	[d]7			[d]7		
BLIM	[d]4								
HMAL	[d]60	88	0.93	33	88	0.91	40	73	0.81
DDAL	6								
HMDG	[d]19	79	0.88	14	86	0.91	15	67	0.79
DDDG	4								

Notes:

[a] For explanation of abbreviations of diagnostic groups, see Table 4.

[b] Number in diagnostic group

[c] % agreed diagnosis out of all those assigned the diagnosis by either rater

[d] N<10: IA_p and kappa not computed

crepancies suggested that items in PSE-10 that describe the clinical course, such as the ICD-10 requirement that delusional symptoms must persist unchanged in the absence of affective symptoms if both are present at some time during an episode, were sometimes not completed or not understood. Such items were subsequently redesigned, and training now emphasises their importance. Only these two categories have a low IA_p; the remaining categories have a very substantial concordance. The indices for Pair 2 were very similar to those for Pair 1.

It is to be expected that congruence would be lower after an interval of time during which the patient's conditions would be likely to change. Delusional psychoses and anxiety states were particularly affected. The other categories with sufficient numbers held their reliability reasonably well (Pair 3).

Concordance between DSM-III-R categories

The concordance on DSM-III-R categories (Table 8.6) was a little lower than for ICD-10, which may be due in part to the confusion noted earlier over the wording of some course criteria. This should be lessened by rewording and attention during training. However, the results in general are much like those for ICD-10.

Agreement between ICD-10 and DSM-III-R categories

Since the two sets of rules use different patterns of items and combine them in different ways, complete concordance between them would not be expected. This is demonstrated in Table 8.7, particularly for the anxiety disorders. For example, F20 data-sets were often classified as 298.9. The numerous course and disability criteria in DSM-III-R contributed much of the variation.

Item group profiles

ICD-10 and DSM-III-R Item Group profiles derived from the PSE-10 data-sets of the field trial interviewer in Pair 1 (see Table 8.4 for mnemonics and Table 8.7 for numbers) are presented for purposes of illustration in Figures 8.1–8.8. They are shown as the percentage of each item group (CATEGO-5) probably or definitely present. The Item Groups then used were numbered from 1–59. A list of these IG names

Table 8.6. Agreement between Pairs on CATEGO-5 DSM-III-R classes

Diagnostic group[a]	Pair 1 Interviewer/Observer			Pair 2 Interviewer/Observer			Pair 3 Int'r/FU		
	N^b	$IA_p{}^c$	Kappa	N	IA_p	K	N	IA_p	K
SZ	81	74	0.82	12	50	0.64	46	63	0.73
SZAF	[d]6								
DL	26	50	0.65	[d]8			18	17	0.25
MNBP	59	63	0.74	14	86	0.91	36	51	0.62
DP	153	73	0.79	27	86	0.90	111	70	0.71
PB	35	63	0.76	[d]9			[d]2		
PNGA	18	50	0.66	[d]6			10	20	0.32
OB	[d]9								
ANEX	[d]6								
BLIM	[d]2								
HMAL	60	82	0.89	[d]			37	81	0.88
DDAL	[d]_								
HMDG	18	79	0.83	[d]			13	46	0.62
DDDG	[d]4								

Notes:

[a] For explanation of mnemonics for diagnostic groups, see Table 4 and Appendix to Chapter 9

[b] Number in diagnostic group

[c] % agreed diagnosis out of all those assigned the diagnosis by either rater

[d] N<10, IA, and kappa not computed

Table 8.7. *Agreement between CATEGO-5 ICD-10 and DSM-III-R classes*

Diagnostic group[a]	Pair 1			Pair 2		
	N[b]	IA$_p$[c]	Kappa	N	IA$_p$	K
SZ	107	67	0.76	19	47	0.61
SZAF	[d]6					
DL	30	60	0.74	15	27	0.38
MNBP	58	64	0.76	16	75	0.84
DP	171	66	0.71	39	64	0.72
PB	32	28	0.42	14	29	0.41
PNGA	20	35	0.51	[d]8		
OB	[d]8					
ANEX	10	40	0.57	[d]7		
BLIM	[d]2					
HMAL	70	79	0.86	37	70	0.78
DDAL	[d]5					
HMDG	24	67	0.79	15	87	0.92
DDDG	[d]6					

Notes:
[a] For explanation of mnemonics for diagnostic groups, see Table 4
[b] Number in diagnostic group
[c] % agreed diagnosis out of all those assigned the diagnosis by either rater
[d] N<10, IA$_p$ and kappa not computed

is provided in Appendix 8.1, because some have changed since then. In spite of the differences in the frequency with which some diagnoses are derived from the same sets of data, the profiles are remarkably similar.

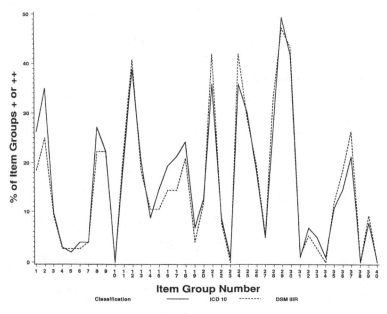

Figure 8.1 Item Group profiles for SZ

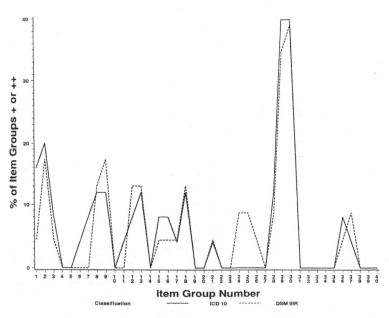

Figure 8.2 Item Group profiles for DL

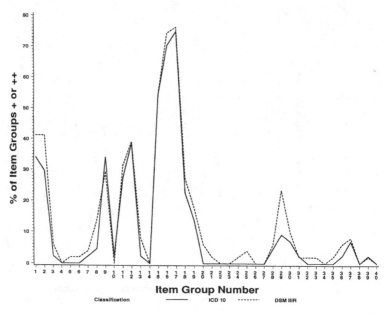

Figure 8.3 Item Group profiles for MNBP

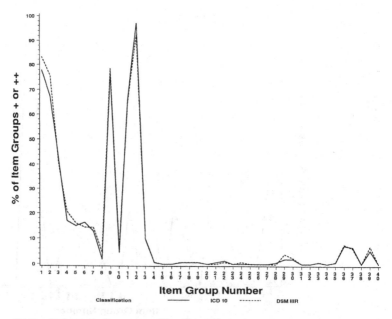

Figure 8.4 Item Group profiles for DP

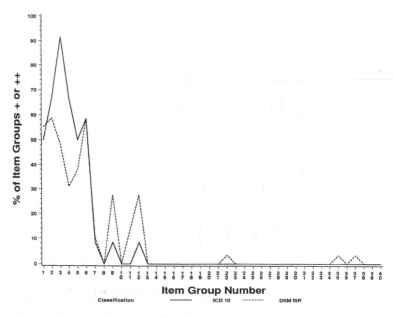

Figure 8.5 Item Group profiles for P B

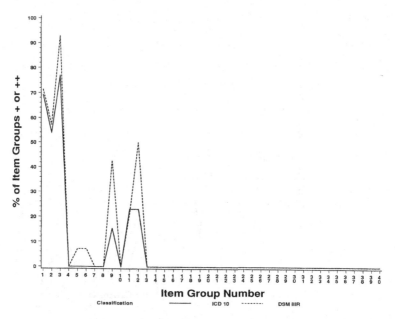

Figure 8.6 Item Group profiles for P N G A

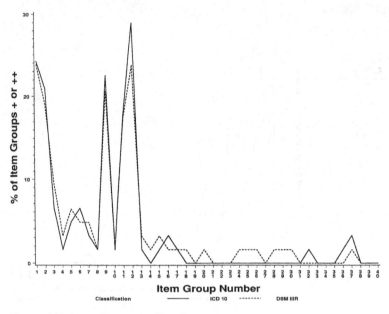

Figure 8.7 Item Group profiles for HMAL

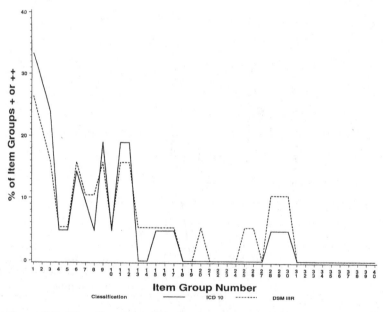

Figure 8.8 Item Group profiles for HMDG

Table 8.8. *Agreement between ST scores; change of score at follow-up*

Symptom Type score	Intraclass correlation		Int'r Pair 1	Int'r Pair 1 minus Int'r Pair 3	
	Pair 1	Pair 2	Mean score	Mean	s.d.
Neurotic	0.96	0.98	15.4	−0.02	8.76
Depressive	0.96	0.97	19.1	−0.02	9.43
Manic	0.98	0.98	3.3	−0.06	3.84
Psychotic	0.98	0.84	4.8	−0.25	6.83
Odd	0.85	*	0.4	0.06	1.31
Negative	0.80	*	1.3	−0.09	2.91
Autistic	0.84	*	*	*	
Substance*					
Eating*					
Cognitive*					

Note:
* Numbers too small or sections not used in trials

Symptom Type (*ST*) scores

Because the wording, order, rating and definition of items in nearly every section changed substantially on the basis of clinical observations during the first field trials and changes in the DCR, kappas for individual items are not presented. Scores based on the summed ratings of similar symptoms, particularly the common ones, should however be robust. Those presented in Table 8.8 are different from those in Table 8.1 because they are based on a later version of the schedule. They subsequently changed again. The intra-class correlations shown in Table 8.8 are high for both Pair 1 and Pair 2 where there were sufficient cases to make a test.

Danish study

A separate study, carried out in Århus, Denmark, included a reliability study of psychotic, affective, anxiety and substance use disorders (Mors and Sørensen, 1993). The results were similar to those of the field trials, but with higher reliability throughout.

Extra testing

A number of extra studies were carried out because of the small number of cases in certain categories derived from the first wave of trials, or because changes in the SCAN rules required substantial changes in the text of subsequent versions of SCAN.

Substance use

Reliability trials of the modified Sections 11 and 12 covering alcohol and other substance use in 10 patients attending specialist services were carried out in SCAN-0 Field Trial Centres (FTCS) in Ankara, Saõ Paulo and Sofia. There was agreement between interviewer and observer on dependence in all but 2 of 29 cases (one could not be included).

Further studies on feasibility and content of the changing sections were carried out in Farmington, Connecticut. Another project, commissioned by NIAAA, was carried out in New York. Thirty people were interviewed twice during July and August 1989, using the alcohol section. They included employees at a medical centre, acquaintances of the five interviewers and four patients. The average time between interviews was 7 days. Four kappas out of 18 items were below 0.5, and these were modified or discarded. There was virtually complete agreement on dependence, harm or no disorder.

Cognitive disorders

The section covering cognitive disorders (now Section 21 in version 2), was not ready in time for the general field trials, but various drafts were later used, without the rest of the SCAN schedules, in three studies in Athens FTC (N 35) and two in Santander FTC (21). There were 114 items in all, including the 35-item MiniMental State (Folstein et al., 1975) and 16 items from CAMDEX (Roth et al., 1986). The five studies were used to develop the section content as well as to test interviewer–observer (N 38) and test-retest (N 20) reliability. New items, scores and Item Groups were developed to cover the problems related to memory, intellect, agnosia and behavioural deterioration listed in the ICD-10 DCR.

The results were very encouraging in the sense that there was very high agreement (Kw = 0.79–0.92) between interviewer and observer on memory, intellectual, global and MiniMental State scores. Agreement on diagnosis of types of dementia (F00-F04 of ICD-10) was also very high (K = 0.86–0.95). Equivalent kappas were reasonably high (0.61–0.67 and 0.86–1.00) in the test-retest group. It should be noted that the diagnostic grouping depends in part on information about physical investigations gathered from the clinical record. This was available to both raters.

Development of SCAN-1

The results of the trials suggested that the feasibility, acceptability and reliability of PSE categories and scores were likely to remain high and would probably improve further. The experience of investigators participating in the field trials was of immense value during the next phase of revision of text and algorithms. ICD-10 had also, meanwhile, moved on, and the draft Diagnostic Criteria for Research for ICD-10 (eventually published definitively in January 1993) provided a further list of items, particularly those concerned with the specification of the course of disorders, that needed to be incorporated.

The development of the algorithms for the first Computer Assisted PSE (CAPSE-1 for PSE-10.1) is described in Chapter 9 because it is part of the history of SCAN and demonstrates the attention to detail that has been characteristic throughout. SCAN-1 was published in April 1992. Events rapidly overtook it, necessitating such substantial revisions that further editions were called for. Important as these changes proved, the main structure and content of SCAN-1 stayed intact in the following versions. SCAN-1 and CAPSE-1 remained in use for some years and further development was based on the experience accumulated during this time. Chapters 10 and 11 then bring the narrative up to date by describing further developments, through SCAN-2.0 to SCAN-2.1/PSE-10.2 and the updated CAPSE-2.

Appendix 8.1   Figures 8.1–8.8   Item group profiles of diagnostic groups SCAN-1

Explanatory notes

1.   The names of the mnemonics of diagnostic groups used in these Figures are listed in Table 8.4.

2. The names of the Item Groups shown in the profiles are listed below. The item-composition (PSE-10, September 1988) of the first 40 did not change substantially after the field trials. IGs from 41 onwards did change a great deal and are not included.
3. The profiles show the average percentage of Item Groups probably or certainly present, by CATEGO-5 diagnostic group. The data are taken from the international field trials.

Item Group names

1. Nervous tension
2. Muscular tension
3. Autonomic anxiety and panic
4. Agoraphobia
5. Social phobias
6. Specific phobias
7. Obsessions and compulsions
8. Depersonalisation etc.
9. Low subjective functioning
10. Low bodily functioning
11. Special depressive symptoms
12. Depressed mood
13. Psychotic depressive symptoms
14. Delusions about the body
15. High subjective functioning
16. Rapid stream of thought
17. Expansive mood
18. Expansive psychotic symptoms
19. Overactivity
20. Odd perceptions
21. Non-specific auditory hallucinations
22. Non-specific visual hallucinations
23. Non-specific psychotic symptoms
24. Non-affective auditory hallucinations
25. Disordered form of thought
26. Replacement of will
27. Bizarre delusions
28. Miscellaneous delusions
29. Delusions of reference

30. Delusions of persecution
31. Emotional liability and turmoil
32. Incoherence of speech
33. Other speech abnormality
34. Socially embarrassing behaviour
35. Flat and incongruous affect
36. Poverty of speech
37. Poor non-verbal communication
38. Self-neglect
39. Psychomotor retardation
40. Catatonic symptoms

References

Bebbington P., Hurry J., Tennant C., Sturt E. and Wing J. K. (1981) The epidemiology of mental disorders in Camberwell. *Psychological Medicine*, 11: 561–80.

Brewin C. R., Wing J. K., Mangran S., Brugha T. and MacCarthy B. (1987) Principles and practice of measuring needs in the long term mentally ill. The MRC Needs for Care Assessment. *Psychological Medicine*, 17: 971–81.

Brewin C. R., Wing J. K., Mangan S., Brugha T., MacCarthy B. and Lesage A. (1987) Needs for care among the long-term mentally ill: A report from the Camberwell High Contact Survey. *Psychological Medicine*, 18: 457–68.

Brewin C. R. and Wing J. K. (1988) *The MRC Needs for Care Assessment manual*. MRC Social Psychiatry Unit, Institute of Psychiatry.

Brugha T. S., Wing J. K., Brewin C. R., MacCarthy B., Mangen S., Lesage A. and Mumford J. (1988) The problems of people in long-term psychiatric day care. An introduction to the Camberwell High Contact Survey. *Psychological Medicine*, 18: 443–56.

Cattell R. B. (1966) The meaning and strategic use of factor analysis. In: Cattell R. B. (ed.) *Handbook of multivariate experimental psychology*. Chicago: Rand McNally.

Cicchetti D. V. and Feinstein A. R. (1990) High agreement but low kappa. II. Resolving the paradoxes. *Journal of Clinical Epidemiology*, 43: 551–8.

Cooper J. E., Copeland J. R. M., Brown G. W., Harris T. and Gourlay A. J. (1977) Further studies on interviewer training and inter-rater reliability of the PSE. *Psychological Medicine*, 7: 517–24.

Cooper J. E., Kendell R. E. Gurland B. J., Sharpe L., Copeland J. R. M. and Simon R. (1972) *Psychiatric diagnoses in New York and London.* London: Oxford University Press.

Folstein M. F., Folstein S. E. and McHugh P. R. (1975) MiniMental State. A practical method for grading the cognitive state of patients for the clinician. *Journal of Psychiatric Research*, 12: 189–98.

Gulbinat W. (1979) Reliability of methods and instruments. In: *Schizophrenia. An international follow-up study*, pp. 61–94. Geneva: WHO.

Isaac M. (1990) SCAN in the third world. In: Stefanis C. N. (ed.) *Psychiatry. A world perspective*, pp. 118–20. Amsterdam: Elsevier.

Kendell R. E., Everett B., Cooper J. E., Sartorius N. and David M. E. (1968) Reliability of the Present State Examination. *Social Psychiatry*, 3: 123–9.

Kreitman N. (1961) Reliability of psychiatric diagnoses. *Journal of Mental Science*, 107: 876.

Luria R. E. and Berry R. (1979) Reliability and descriptive validity of the PSE syndromes. *Archives of General Psychiatry*, 36: 1187–95.

Luria R. E. and McHugh P. (1974) Reliability and clinical utility of the 'Wing' PSE. *Archives of General Psychiatry*, 30: 866–71.

Mavreas V. G., Vazquez-Barquero J. L., Kontaxakis V., Ploumbidis D. (1990) Diagnosing dementias with the SCAN. In: Stefanis C. N. (ed.) *Psychiatry. A world perspective*, vol. I, pp. 113–17. Amsterdam: Elsevier.

Maxwell A. E. (1977) Coefficients of agreement between observers, and their interpretation. *British Journal of Psychiatry*, 130: 79–83.

McGuffin P., Katz R. and Aldrich J. (1986) Past and present state examination. The assessment of 'lifetime ever' psychopathology. *Psychological Medicine* 16: 461–6.

Mors O. and Sørensen L. V. (1993) Incidence and co-morbidity of psychiatric disorders from a well-defined catchment area in Denmark. *European Psychiatry*, 8: 193–9.

Pakaslahti A. (1987) Applicability and reliability of the PSE in a Finnish study. *Psychiatrica Fennica*, 18: 63–72.

Rogers S. B. and Mann S. A. (1986) The reliability and validity of PSE assessments by lay interviewers. A national population survey. *Psychological Medicine*, 16: 689–700.

Roth M., Tym B., Mountjoy C. Q., Huppert F. A., Hendrie H., Verma S. and Goddard R. (1986) CAMDEX. A standardised instrument for the diagnosis of mental disorder in the elderly with special reference to the early detection of dementia. *British Journal of Psychiatry* 149: 698–709.

Sturt E., Bebbington P., Hurry J. and Tenneant C. (1981) The PSE used by interviewers from a survey agency. *Psychological Medicine*, 11: 185–92.

Tomov T. and Nikolov V. (1990) Reliability of SCAN categories and scores.

Results of the field trials. In: Stefanis C. N. (ed.) *Psychiatry. A world perspective*, vol. I, pp. 107–12. Amsterdam: Elsevier.

Üstün T. B. (1990) SCAN: ICD-10 and DSM-III-R diagnoses. In: Stefanis C. N. (ed.) *Psychiatry. A world perspective*, vol. I, pp. 100–6. Amsterdam: Elsevier.

Wing J. K. (1990) Introduction to the field trials of SCAN. In: Stefanis C. N. (ed.) *Psychiatry. A world perspective*, pp. 91–2. Amsterdam: Elsevier.

Wing J. K., Birley J. L. T., Cooper J. E., Graham P. and Isaacs A. (1967) Reliability of a procedure for measuring and classifying 'present psychiatric state'. *British Journal of Psychiatry*, 113: 499–515.

Wing J. K., Cooper J. E. and Sartorius N. (1974) *The measurement and classification of psychiatric symptoms*. London: Cambridge University Press.

Wing J. K., Nixon J. M., Mann S. A. and Leff J. P. (1977) Reliability of the PSE (ninth edition) used in a population survey. *Psychological Medicine*, 7: 505–516.

Wing J. K., Mann S. A., Leff J. P. and Nixon J. M. (1978) The concept of a 'case' in psychiatric population surveys. *Psychological Medicine*, 8: 203–17.

Wing J. K. and Sturt E. (1978) *The PSE-ID-CATEGO system. A supplementary manual (mimeograph)*. London: MRC Social Psychiatry Unit.

World Health Organization (1973) *The international pilot study of schizophrenia*. Geneva: WHO.

World Health Organization (1980) *International classification of impairments, disabilities and handicaps*. Geneva: WHO.

Zubin J. (1967) Classification of the behaviour disorders. *Annual Review of Psychology*, 18: 373–401.

9 SCAN-1: Algorithms and CAPSE-1

G. Der, G. Glover, T. S. Brugha and J. K. Wing

Introduction

It has been accepted, in Chapter 1, that the ICD-10 term, 'mental disorder' is more appropriate than the term 'disease' in the present state of development of psychiatric nosology. Until biological markers are as well established as, for example, in diabetes, research of all kinds – biological, psychological and social – is likely to be fostered by the development of clinical assessment systems that allow clinical phenomena (experiential and behavioural) to be elicited, recognised and recorded reliably. This provides a basis of clinical fact broad enough, and defined and described in terms specific enough, to allow world-wide communicability, irrespective of classification.

The application of sets of classifying rules to this database is, relatively speaking, a simpler problem, although it tends to be the one that most workers think of first when trying to standardise methods of diagnosis. They start with the classifying criteria, and are well satisfied if these can be specified, in terms of rules linking clinical items delineated only by their names, clearly and simply enough to be easily used in practice by most clinicians. The strategy is least effective when there are many different sets of such rules, with rather little in the way of empirical validation for any one of them. A sensible solution is to adopt one or two of them (e.g. ICD-10 and DSM-IV) as standard, or reference, sets. If the database is broad enough, research workers can use, in addition, whatever other classifications suit their purpose.

The output of the SCAN system, therefore, can be as simple or as complex as any of its users require, if they are able and willing to analyse the material collected themselves. Most users, however, want a standard output that will serve many functions reasonably well. Experience in the field trials of SCAN-0 demonstrated that the following output functions were regarded as important:

- ICD-10, DSM-III-R, and eventually DSM-IV, category profiles with episode dates
- Index of Definition for ICD-10 (*ID*)
- Item Group (*IG*) probabilities, score profile and rating table
- Symptom Type (*ST*) score profile
- List of items rated present
- Standard statistical analysis of data from a series of cases
- PSE-10/PSE-9 conversion with output from CATEGO-4

Creating the diagnostic algorithms

At that time DSM-III-R (1987) and ICD-10 provided lists of operational rules for making diagnoses. For ICD-10, these took the form of Diagnostic Criteria for Research (DCR). Several versions were published during the course of the field trials, and the designers of SCAN were therefore presented with a moving target. Both the text of the SCAN schedule and the algorithms had to be adapted in order to take account of changes, at the same time as ensuring sufficient stability to enable the trials to take place. The version of CAPSE-1 to be described was compatible with the DCR available in July 1992. The definitive DCR were not published until January 1993, and the further changes required are described, together with those for DSM-IV, in Chapters 10 and 11.

Some of the problems of translating seemingly clear-cut rules into SCAN items and CAPSE algorithms, while preserving clinical meaning, have been discussed in Chapters 2 and 3. We are concerned here with ways of solving the technical problems. The issues are similar for the two diagnostic systems, so ICD-10 will be used to illustrate the solutions that were adopted.

The early algorithms for PSE-9 were written in a concocted logical language (CATEGO-3, published as Chapter 6 of the instruction manual, Wing, Cooper and Sartorius, 1974; later slightly modified as CATEGO-4, Wing and Sturt, 1978). This was translated into Fortran for batch processing. A similar procedure was followed for CATEGO-5. The initial algorithms were written in SPSS for ICD-9 for the prototype SCAN (1 September 1983). Following the first unofficial DCR these were modified and coded in SAS. This resulted in the version used in the field trials (CATEGO-5; Chapter 8).

As Centres returned their data, including the hospital diagnoses, collaborators made detailed comments on a wide range of issues relating to the practical use of SCAN and the meaning of the output returned to them. Meanwhile frequent changes were being made to the ICD-10 rules (official versions April 1989, February 1990, May 1990 and finally January 1993). It became clear that the process of revising the SCAN text and algorithms would be piecemeal, lengthy and tedious. However, the task was eased considerably, and made more interesting, by the use of an expert system.

The expert system

The expert system was a computerised program for writing and testing algorithms. A straightforward 'if–then' logic, expressed in a simplified and standardised near-English, applied the rules specified in the DCR to the data recorded in PSE-10 or the Item Group Checklist. The system could be used either to write and change the classifying algorithm, or to apply it to a set of data, e.g. one of the cases sent in from the Field Trial Centres. By switching between these two modes, the algorithm could be developed and updated in a very flexible way. Any part of the algorithm could rapidly be inspected, altered, tested against real data and then further developed and re-tested. Only simple programming skills and computer expertise were required.

The system could only be used to process one set of data at a time; it was not intended for batch processing. Also, it was not simple to incorporate exclusion rules, which were generally left for a subsequent round of programming. The central advantage of the system was that it allowed points in the program where clinical decisions should be made to be readily identified, solved, entered, tested and, if necessary, further modified. Composing new sections of the algorithm was relatively painless. The maximum advantage was gained by a combination of expert system with conventional programming.

While the expert system approach was well suited to the process of developing algorithms, the computer implementation of the developed algorithm had different requirements. It was more important that the production programs be portable, compact and efficient – qualities which were not so important in the developing system and which the expert system used largely lacked. The calculation of scores would have required enhancements to the expert system. Finally, the expert system was geared to interactive operation on a case-by-case basis, whereas the production programs need the ability to process batches of interviews in a non-interactive fashion.

The algorithms developed using the expert system were therefore translated and expanded using the 'C' programming language. This was chosen for its portability across a wide range of computers and operating systems and to provide comparability with other WHO/ADAMHA algorithms, e.g. those for CIDI. C programs can be difficult to read, largely because the language allows very terse expressions to be constructed. However, in writing the diagnostic programs, the policy has been to keep it simple; the readability of the code was given higher priority than conciseness or efficiency. This applied particularly to the sections that embody the diagnostic algorithm. The aim was to produce a code that a non-programmer could understand with minimal help.

Computer assisted administration of SCAN: CAPSE-1

The recent development of powerful computers that are both readily portable and comparatively cheap has made computer-based administration of rating instruments a realistic possibility. This offers several advantages for SCAN:

1. Storage of results on magnetic disc is far more compact than on paper. Copies can readily be made for storage in different locations for security purposes. The process of transcription from paper to computer for analysis is avoided; saving time, money and transcription errors.

2. With ingenuity, the printed interview and Glossary text have been made usable in clinical situations, but moving from section to section and question to question remains complicated until the system has been fully learned. Computerisation simplifies the process of moving about the instrument and makes relevant Glossary entries available at a single keystroke.

3. The Glossary definitions are incorporated into help screens so that examiners can consult them rapidly when needed during an interview rather than having to look them up in the manual.

4. Data entry at the time of interview allows for immediate analysis using the suite of programs that provide ICD-10 and DSM-III-R classifications. This may be of use in research settings where the choice of subsequent rating instruments depends on the outcome of the SCAN interview. It is also likely to prove useful in training settings,

where the performance of several trainees in rating a single case can be analysed. Finally it may make the instrument interesting to practising clinicians for use as a standard part of the diagnostic evaluation of in-patients.

5. Similar considerations suggest that it would be useful to add an option for a routine statistical analysis of a series of cases entered into a computer file as the interviews were conducted, so that comparisons could be made between series collected at the same or different sites.

Use of the equivalent implementation by Gyles Glover for PSE-9, and extensive use of the first computer-assisted version for PSE-10 (CAPSE-1, July 1992), suggested that most patients found the procedure acceptable, at least in areas where computers were commonly used.

Design considerations in computerisation

In designing the computer implementation, it was assumed that the IBM PC standard configuration would be most appropriate, and that many users would need a system that worked on the most basic IMB PCs available. The system therefore made no use of colour, graphic facilities or mouse. It was also assumed that the system should allow all the features open to users of the pen and paper version. The most obvious feature incorporated for this purpose was the 'notebook', which allowed the user to make free text comments. These were linked to the question currently being addressed and stored in the main data file.

In designing the environment for the interviewer, care was taken to allow both for novice and for experienced users. A tree-like structure was available for those who were learning to move about the system. Experienced users could jump to specified items simply by typing in the section and item numbers.

The program was written to be as independent as possible of the text that appeared on screen in order to allow translation into other languages. The feasibility of non-English versions was limited only by the availability of screen character drivers for IBM PC compatible computers.

Output from SCAN-1

The output from the programs took two forms. The standard output was in the form of a brief report showing the *ST* scores and total score, the diagnoses (with dates), as well as respondent numbers and a few sociodemographic items. The ICD-10 or DSM-III-R diagnoses were given both as codes and names, separately for each episode, together with dates. The report could be viewed on screen or directed to a file. More detailed reports were available as options.

The second form of output was designed to be read into other programs. This was produced automatically and stored in a file containing diagnostic codes, item groups and their scores plus identifying information and some sociodemographic items. The data were in a fixed format and could easily be read into a standard statistical package for further analysis.

An offshoot of this work was a preliminary study of a computer-conducted interview based on SCAN-1 (Brugha et al., 1996).

References

Brugha T. S., Kaul A., Dignon A., Teather D. and Wills K. M. (1996) Present State Examination by microcomputer. Objective and experience of preliminary steps. *International Journal of Methods in Psychiatric Research*, 6: 1–9.

Wing J. K., Cooper J. E. and Sartorius N. (1974) *The measurement and classification of psychiatric symptoms. An instruction manual for the PSE and CATEGO program.* London: Cambridge University Press.

Wing J. K. and Sturt E. (1978) *The PSE-ID-CATEGO system. A supplementary manual.* London: MRC Social Psychiatry Unit, Institute of Psychiatry.

10   Development of SCAN-2.1

T. S. Brugha

Reasons for modification

The development and printing of SCAN-1/PSE-10.1 is mentioned briefly at the end of Chapter 8. The following account of the changes incorporated during the revision for SCAN-2.0 and then SCAN-2.1/PSE-10.2 is presented both for the record and for the benefit of those familiar with SCAN-1.

Preliminary experience with sections first incorporated in SCAN-1 highlighted the need for a number of further changes. Section 2 (Physical Health, Somatoform and Dissociative Disorder) needed to cover more accurately and clearly the classification rules of DSM-III-R and ICD-10. Similarly, users of Sections 11 and 12 (Alcohol and Psychoactive Substances) had encountered difficulties and some had found the length of the sections unnecessarily tedious. Users of Section 20 (Cognitive Impairment and/or Decline) also generated detailed suggestions. While it was recognised that Section 20 was designed as a screening tool, desire for greater diagnostic information was also expressed. SCAN and PSE users who were not familiar with the concepts of Acute Stress Reaction and Adjustment Disorder (Section 1) also called for clarification.

The introduction in SCAN-1, in rating scale I, of the '6' rating ('symptom present but physical illness makes rating difficult) and '7' (trait rating) was also criticised. Trainers and interviewers expressed a concern that it could be difficult to know whether to rate a symptom present (2 or 3), a trait (7), or a physical cause (6). Moreover, a rating of 6 did not allow severity to be included. A group in Baltimore (Anthony et al., 1985) had begun to develop a clinical assessment method based on an extension of PSE-9, in which the examiner was required to record separately a clinical judgement as to whether a symptom was due to an external substance or to physical ill health. The view was that the record of such attributions should be separate from rating scale I. This matter is discussed later.

However, the most compelling reasons for producing first SCAN-

2.0 and then SCAN-2.1 were last minute changes in the final published version of the ICD-10 Diagnostic Criteria for Research (DCR; WHO, 1993), and some changes needed for extra coverage of a few areas of DSM-III-R, and the introduction of DSM IV in May 1994 (APA, 1994). During the final intensive period of programming CAPSE-2 (see Chapter 11) a detailed analysis of the complete algorithms for ICD-10 and DSM-4 demonstrated a large number of relatively small but important differences between concepts with the same or similar names. Finalisation of the text had to be delayed until SCAN advisors were satisfied that the clinical concepts of both systems were properly covered. This chapter lists only the major changes incorporated into the final text of SCAN-2.1/PSE-10.2 and the CAPSE-2 software.

Structure of SCAN-2.1

The overall structure of SCAN-2 (see Appendix to Chapter 3) differs very little from that of SCAN version 1. The distinction between the two versions is assisted by the introduction of a new style of item numbering. As before, the Section number (now 0–27) appears on the left of the decimal point. But item numbers are now all 3-digit. Thus item 3.1 in SCAN-1 has become 3.001 in SCAN-2.1. The checklists for Acute Stress Reaction and Adjustment Disorders were moved from Section 1 (SCAN-1) to Section 13 (SCAN-2.1). Section 13 was enlarged further with the inclusion of ratings of attributions of cause and of the hierarchical relationship between Part One symptoms and syndromes. Section 19 (SCAN-1) was subdivided into two sections. This division was interposed after item 19.47 in v1 (Identify Organic Cause of Section 19 Symptoms). A new section, numbered Section 20 in SCAN-2.1, begins, therefore, with the item 'Length of Episode of Schizophrenia'. In addition to the various checklists that had been included in Section 19 (SCAN-1), the new Section 20 (version 2) includes an optional series of items for rating Attributions of Cause in Part Two and, at the end of the section, a checklist for negative syndrome items. This optional checklist was included for research purposes. Similarly, the final section on Clinical History (CHS) became Section 27 in SCAN-2.1.

The most substantial structural change is due to the enhanced sections at the end of Part One (Section 13) and the corresponding point in Part Two (Section 20). Both provide an opportunity to review and make summary ratings of the preceding sections of the interview. By allowing users of SCAN-2.1 to delay until the end of Part One and

Part Two decisions about attributions of cause and about reasons for interference with activities, it is envisaged that the examiner's task will be simpler and less interrupted. Most sections now provide an option for rating two periods. Section 2 (Somatoform items) also now requires ratings of the two years before the examination.

Additions to the item pool

Interference with activities; timing of symptoms

SCAN-2 retains the comprehensive, bottom-up clinical assessment characteristics of its predecessors. An important enhancement, now included in most sections, is a set of ratings of 'Interference with activities' and of 'Period timing'. Thus, in Sections 13 and 20, and at least once and sometimes more than once in each preceding section, the examiner can now rate interference with activities due to items in that section. The rating of interference with day-to-day activities *due* to a symptom should not be confused with the concept of interference with functioning inherent in the rating of most PSE symptoms (see Introduction to Rating Scales I and II). Of particular use is the opportunity to record the onset of the Present State/Present Episode Period and, if chosen, the Onset and Recovery Date of a previous Representative Episode or Lifetime Before Period of symptoms in the section. This enhancement could be useful in cases, for example, of Depressive Episode (*PS/PE*) in respondents who also describe neurotic symptoms such as obsessional or anxiety symptoms with a significantly different time course. For example, some specific phobias can be dated by respondents back to early childhood. This record would clearly delineate such long-standing neurotic disorders from a more recent episode for example, of depression. The reliability of these new ratings will need to be carefully assessed. Trait ratings are now optionally available in a separate attributional rating scale (see below), and not as in rating scale I of version 1.

Changes to Sections derived from PSE-9

Anxiety items

In revising Section 4 on anxiety, it was recognised that the distinction between Somatoform Disorders and Anxiety Disorders, in both of which numerous somatic symptoms may be described by respondents, can give rise to confusion. An extra instruction was inserted into Section 4 to remind the examiner to consider the need to use the somatoform checklists in Section 2. A number of alterations to the Anxiety symptom checklist were required for classification purposes and, as discussed later in the chapter, to clarify the distinction between DSM and ICD-10 concepts and definitions of anxiety. Most of these changes were achieved by modifying the existing items. New items include 4.016 'Feeling of Choking'. Another new item in Section 4 is item 4.021, 'Enduring Apprehension of Having Another Panic Attack'. As in other sections, new items dealing with Interference and Timing were introduced, but in Section 4 separate ratings of Avoidance and Interference were introduced for each of the three types of phobia.

Obsessional items

Apart from several items dealing with interrelationships between obsessional and non-obsessional items, two items were added to Section 5: 5.011, 'Insight into Obsessional Symptoms' and 5.012, 'Content of Obsessional Symptoms Limited to Another Disorder'. The inclusion in section 5 of a separate dating of the Period or Periods of Section 5 symptoms is expected to be particularly useful, as the onset of some obsessional phenomena can be dated by respondents back to childhood.

Mood items, Sections 6, 7, 8 and 10

The decision to modify item 6.1 'Depressed Mood' in version 1, in order to incorporate a record of duration of the affect, was reconsidered. In SCAN-2.1, item 6.001 reverted to its original form (in PSE-9, item 23) with the rating of 'Depressed Mood' to be used with rating scale I only. A PSE-9 item, 'Social Withdrawal', which had not been included in previous versions of PSE-10, was reintroduced into version 2.1 as item 6.016.

Various other changes required for DSM-IV were introduced. The checklist of 'Persistent Depressive State' items was extended. Each checklist item now includes cross-references to the corresponding item numbers elsewhere in SCAN-2.1. The dating of previous, or recent, episodes of 'Depressive Disorder' before the present episode (PE) was introduced to deal with seasonal, rapid cycling and other

recurrent episodes. The decision to record dates rather than to intro-
duce additional ratings of the number, type and interrelationship of
previous episodes, means that data gathered using v2 should continue
to be useful if and when classification rules for recurrent forms of
'Affective Disorder' undergo changes in future. Within Section 8,
items on 'Weight' and 'Sleep' were more clearly separated from items
on problems with 'Sex'. Users can now record dates and interference
separately within these two parts of Section 8.

A method for assessing psychosexual dysfunction has not been
developed. However, an instruction is included following the three
Sexual Dysfunction items, that refers to the optional use of a new
ICD-10 DCR checklist of psychosexual problems, included in the
Clinical History Schedule. Some clarifications have also been introduced to Section 9 on 'Eating Disorders'. In Section 10, on
'Expansive Mood', most items are now rated independently of time
duration, a possible source of confusion introduced in the first
version of SCAN. There is a separate new item for 'Duration of
Expansive or Irritable Mood', 10.003. 'Irritable Mood', 10.002, is
new. Other changes to Section 10 are similar to the changes introduced into Section 6, providing detailed information on dates of
earlier periods of affective symptoms.

Changes to Sections that were new in SCAN-1

Somatoform and dissociative symptoms (Physical Health)

The aim of the editors has been to clarify terminology and aid practical use. An important enhancement, already referred to under
anxiety items, is provided at the beginning and end of this section.
Users are advised to be aware that somatic and anxiety symptoms
may present in similar ways. At the end of the section a new item,
'Relationship between Somatoform and Anxiety Symptoms', has
been inserted, together with a cross-reference to Section 4.

Use of alcohol and psychoactive substances

Numerous changes have been made to these two sections, principally
in order to deal with enhancements to ICD-10 DCR and to DSM-IV.
Some changes have also been introduced following experience gained
in cross-cultural field studies with SCAN-1. The estimation of quan-

tity of alcohol intake has been simplified, and the item 11.14, 'Cultural Attitude to Alcohol', deleted. More detailed information on the relationship between mental-health problems and use of both alcohol and psychoactive substances is now incorporated in SCAN-2.1. Both polymorphic and mixed presentation of symptoms can also be recorded.

Cognitive impairment

Although still a screening device for use as part of a general examination the diagnostic capabilities of this section have been extended. The original MiniMental State examination now appears above the section cut-off. In revising this section (Section 20 in version 1) it was recognised that some difficulties could be encountered by users in different cultures, particularly with elderly respondents who had not had the opportunity of attending formal schooling. A new item, the 'Verbal Trails Test', Item 21.002, could not be utilised in its existing form in such settings. Section 21 (version 2) has also been organised into subsections with some considerable reordering of items compared with Version 1. The sections cover memory, remote memory, language, calculation, praxis, abstraction, fund of knowledge, frontal subcortical tests and level of consciousness. Sections on 'Overall Ratings of Cognitive Impairment' and of 'Recent Clinical History' are as they appeared in SCAN-1.

Stress and adjustment attributions

The 'Stress and Adjustment Disorder' optional checklists have been moved from their earlier location at the end of Section 1 in SCAN-1 to Section 13 at the end of Part One of SCAN-2. Most stress and adjustment disorder symptoms appear initially in Sections 3 and 4, and some appear also in the sections covering Depression. Examiners might not have been in a position to judge whether symptoms could be directly linked, temporally, to external stressors until these earlier sections had been fully covered. It should now be more straightforward for examiners to make judgements of such attributions. The examiner begins by rating possible causes, adverse events or circumstances in items 13.050 through to 13.058. Detailed information can now be recorded concerning the time course of symptoms for 'Acute Reactions', 'Delayed Post Traumatic Stress Reactions' and

'Adjustment Disorders', going beyond the required classification rules and adding to the descriptive bottom-up data range of SCAN.

Attribution of causes

Rating of attributions in earlier versions

The '6' rating in rating scale I of SCAN-1 gave rise to difficulties, as reported earlier (see Reasons for Modification at the head of this chapter). Items *should* be rated on presence and severity, independently of the possible influence of an external cause, whether due to physical illness or a substance or medication. This is catered for in SCAN-1 and -2.1 by including an appropriate item at the end of each relevant section. It might therefore be argued that an equivalent item should be included to cover psychogenic, social and treatment influences. To some extent these are catered for in Section 1 of SCAN-2.1 (Psychosocial Interventions), and as discussed above for Sections 13 and 20.

Top-down and bottom-up solutions and implementation for testing

Optional solutions to the problem of attributional ratings are available in SCAN-2.1. Judgements of attributions require experience and skills in medicine and clinical pharmacology and related areas. Examiners not so qualified can opt not to use the scales. There are three types of option:

1. At an individual item level, users can now rate the influence of treatments, alcohol and psychoactive substances, intracranial processes, toxins and medication, in dashed boxes below the standard rating boxes. The option is available in the text only as appropriate, e.g. at item 2.084, 'Hypochrondriacal Preoccupation'.
2. At the end of each section and sometimes within sections, there is an opportunity to rate organic cause of symptoms and to record the ICD-10 code for the influence or cause of those symptoms. This is very similar to the 'organic cause' option available in SCAN-1.
3. There is also an opportunity to rate these and other attributions in Sections 13 and 20 instead. In Sections 13 and 20 users may record the quality of data available when rating such attributions. Users may also either record or modify previous attributional ratings within earlier sections of SCAN. Similar records can be made at the end of Part One, in Section 13, and in Part Two in Section 20.

The stringent ICD-10 criteria for rating attributions of cause are listed on pages 180–90 and 260 of the interview. The implications and possible pitfalls involved in attempting to separate 'organic' from 'functional' mental disorders have been considered by Lewis (1994) and Henderson et al. (1994) in relation to ICD-10, and will be of relevance to the increased prominence of this topic in DSM-IV.

SCAN-2 Glossary

Few changes to the SCAN-1 Glossary were required in order to produce version 2.1. Definitions for the few new items were added, with appropriate rating instructions. Occasionally, the earlier definitions were updated in minor ways, based on additional cross-references designed to clarify distinctions between similar items.

Revised classification rules and SCAN-2

ICD-10 final draft of DCR after field trials

SCAN-1 has been used extensively, with the ICD-10 DCR, in clinical research, in community surveys and in the national psychiatric morbidity surveys in Great Britain (Melzer et al., 1995). The field trials of the DCR led to a limited number of detailed modifications to the rules for various diagnoses. The final published draft of the DCR (WHO, 1993) was compared with the earlier field trial version and the necessary changes identified.

Only one major set of modifications appeared to be required. The 'Psychoactive Substance Use' section of the DCR, in its final version, is a great deal more detailed, with specific listings of toxic symptoms caused by substances and of symptoms arising in withdrawal states. Most of the necessary symptoms were already listed in the SCAN-1 Glossary, and relatively minor modifications were required in order to bring the instrument up to date. The only other section of SCAN requiring more than minimal change was the 'Anxiety Section' where a number of additional symptoms in the checklist, together with modifications of existing symptoms, were required. There were no major changes in the 'Affective Disorders' (F3) nor in the 'Non-Organic Psychoses' (F2). Once again the bottom-up design of the Present State Examination has proved to be surprisingly future-proof and robust. A further difficulty, not specified clearly in SCAN-1, was the requirement to record the co-occurrence of anxiety symptoms within a spell or attack. This is now incorporated into the modified rating scale for the symptom checklist in Section 4.

DSM IV

Numerous modifications were required in the light of the fourth edition of the APA Diagnostic and Statistical Manual (DSM-IV). This provided editors with an opportunity to recheck the coverage of the earlier DSM-III-R and to attend to gaps. DSM-IV has more specific requirements for disorders due to general medical conditions, hence the increased importance of ratings of records of attributions of physical cause. However, this does not remove the obligation on investigators to assess the clinical validity of such attributions.

Diagnostic criteria for 'Anxiety Disorders'

While producing SCAN-2.1, it was recognised that a distinction between ICD-10 and the DSM series had not been adequately taken into account in earlier versions. In ICD-10, 'Anxiety Disorders' cannot be diagnosed unless 'Autonomic Symptoms' ('Heart Pounding, Missing Beats, Faster'; 'Sweating, e.g. Palms'; 'Trembling or Shaking e.g. of Hands or Limbs'; 'Dry Mouth Not Due To Medication or Dehydration') are clearly present. In DSM-III-R and DSM-IV it is possible to diagnose generalised anxiety disorder in the absence of autonomic symptoms. The Phobia Checklist Rating Scale in SCAN-2 has therefore been modified to take account of this contingency.

Affective disorders

The modifications required have been described earlier. An increased interest, notably in DSM-IV, in the episodic nature of the course of affective disorders is now more comprehensively covered in Sections 6 and 10 of SCAN-2.1.

Substance use

The alterations in Sections 11 and 12 are detailed and many. They include an item to cover legal consequences of alcohol or substance use.

Prodromal and negative features of schizophrenia

Some specific classification requirements of DSM-III-R, in particular the active, prodromal and residual phases of episodes of schizophrenia are included in item 20.001, 'Length of Episode of Schizophrenia', with cross referencing to negative symptom items in Sections 22 to 24. An optional checklist has been added at the end of Section 20 – 'Negative Syndrome' listing items 20.089 through to 20.112. As for all new sections and checklists in SCAN, users proposing to try out these items should first establish whether it is possible to assess and rate them reliably.

Short form of PSE-10

A form of PSE-10 has been prepared by Aksel Bertelsen for use by clinicians. It consists only of symptom items specified in the DCR for ICD-10. A Danish A5 spiral-bound pocket version has been tried out, together with the pocket-book version of ICD-10, with satisfactory results. The English edition is available from Dr Bertelsen, Århus Psychiatric Hospital, DK-8240 Risskov, Denmark.

Conclusions

The need for field testing

The importance of field testing new items, checklists and sections has been emphasised several times throughout this volume. Testing in different languages, societies, cultural groupings and geographic settings is particularly valuable. Many of the changes to SCAN during the revision process have emerged from such studies. SCAN-2.1 will now require another round of testing.

Implications for training

Very few SCAN users are now sufficiently familiar with the whole instrument to be confident of training others in all details. But training sessions are themselves a source of new suggestions for improvement, particularly those that lead to improved clarity in items, rules and concepts. A new round of training (including training the trainers) is now taking place.

Translations

The revisions of SCAN have been fully documented in a series of for-matted computer entered text files. Copies can be obtained from the World Health Organization Division of Mental Health. Translators, and others interested in a detailed comparison of the various drafts and versions of SCAN, will be able to highlight differences using document comparison facilities available in their word processors. These should prove useful to those who have already completed trans-lations of SCAN Version 1 and wish to make the necessary changes for Version 2. Those who are new to the process of translation should take account of the extensive literature and advice and previous expe-rience available on the changes involved in translating such material (see Chapter 5).

Publication of the SCAN-2.1 Interview Manual

The final text of the interview manual for SCAN-2.1, including PSE-10.2 with an updated Item Group Checklist (IGC-2) and Clinical History Schedule (CHS-2), is published together with this reference manual.

References

American Psychiatric Association (1987) *Diagnostic and statistical manual of mental disorders*, third edition revised. Washington DC: APA.

American Psychiatric Association (1994) *Diagnostic and statistical manual of mental disorders*, fourth edition. Washington DC: APA.

Anthony J. C., Folstein M., Romanoski A. J. et al. (1985) Comparison of the lay diagnostic interview schedule and a standardised psychiatric diagno-sis. *Archives of General Psychiatry*, 42: 667–75.

Henderson S., Jablensky A. and Sartorius N. (1994) ICD-10: A neuropsychi-atrist's nightmare? *British Journal of Psychiatry*, 165: 273–5.

Lewis S. (1994) ICD-10: A neuropsychiatrist's nightmare? *British Journal of Psychiatry*, 164: 157–9.

Melzer H., Gill B., Pettigrew M. and Hinds K. (1995) *OPCS surveys of psychiatric morbidity in Great Britain. Report 1. The prevalence of psychi-*

atric morbidity among adults living in private households. London: OPCS Social Survey Division.

World Health Organisation (1992) *SCAN: Schedules for clinical assessment in neuropsychiatry*. Geneva: WHO.

World Health Organization (1993) *ICD-10*, chapter F, Mental and behavioural disorders, diagnostic criteria for research. Geneva: WHO.

11 Computerisation of SCAN-2.1: CAPSE-2

A. Y. Tien, S. Chatterji, and T. B. Üstün

Introduction

The diagnostic process in psychiatry has traditionally relied on gathering information through individual history-taking and clinical examination. When operationalising the concepts involved in order to be able to exploit the opportunities offered by computers it is important to understand clearly what their advantages and disadvantages are compared with human beings (Conrad, 1993). Humans are unmatched in pattern recognition, decision-making and clinical administration. Computers excel at repetitive and conceptually trivial tasks such as recording and retrieving numbers and text, and can provide high-speed analyses of the relationships between data. The development of comprehensive systems to aid the systematic and reliable collection of clinical data, to which specific algorithms can be applied to ensure the comparability of classifications, has been described in earlier chapters. Instruments such as SCAN, CIDI and IPDE are the most recent and complete examples. The three key components that current computer technology provides are database, graphical display and multimedia recording and playback function (Dittman, 1991; Sartorius et al., 1993; Üstün and Tien, 1995). These are summarised below and expanded later in the chapter.

Database: SCAN allows complex data interactions to be recorded, e.g. between defined clinical symptoms, their severity and their time relationships, thus facilitating further refinements and developments.

Graphics: Human abilities in pattern recognition and decision-making can be substantially enhanced by employing computers to display information from the database graphically. For example, a chart showing longitudinal data from repeated assessments of a patient can reveal patterns of temporal association between specific symptoms of depression and varying levels of alcohol misuse. Graphical display of this information can be useful, not only to the clinician, but also for the patient. The computer can also display the structural details of the algorithms, facilitating more widespread understanding and further developments of consensus.

Multi media facilities: Training interviewers and ensuring reliability is enhanced by the use of audio or video recordings. Computer digital recording of an interview allows faster access to playback portions of the interview for reliability study. The digital recordings are a resource for developing education and training materials, helping to improve standardisation of the SCAN internationally. The clinical use of SCAN with computer digital recording also has longer-term implications for medical records and quality assurance. Routine clinical use of a computerised version of SCAN would provide an important link between clinical activities and assessment and a worldwide database supporting a real-time clinical psychiatric epidemiology (Tien, 1994).

Development of the SCAN Version 2.1 application

Ease of use

The use of computers as clinical tools has been increasing rapidly, and patients are becoming familiar with computers as part of the routine clinical environment. The use of computers with and by patients is not generally problematic. It is still uncommon to find professionals using computers while interviewing, but it is feasible to expect that most will eventually do so. Providing a computerised SCAN that is easy to understand and simple to use will facilitate acceptance by clinicians. Ease of use requires speed, simplicity, consistency, familiarity, attractiveness, modifiability, upgradeability and versatility.

Structured or semi-structured interviews are often perceived by clinicians as being lengthy, laborious and monotonous. Time is of the essence. The interview must balance comprehensiveness and utility. Computerisation minimises the time spent relative to the data gathered, and makes the best use of the material without further substantial delay. The clinician must also be able to make rapid checks of diagnostic maps to find a match (or mismatch) between a clinical diagnosis and diagnosis generated by algorithm. This is an important means of refining clinical skills.

Clinicians should not feel restrained by the structure, or feel that their spontaneous approach to information gathering is hampered and therefore inefficient. The PSE interview is highly flexible (see Chapter 4) and the computerised version must allow the clinician to move back and forth in the interview rapidly, check definitions, rating scales, dates, criteria etc., and refer easily to earlier profiles of the same respondent. There should be an opportunity to record observations other than item ratings and to make notes while the interview is in progress. It must also be possible to store unfinished interviews for later completion.

The SCAN computer application requirement includes the flexibility for modification as the instruments are updated and to take advantage of advances in technology, for example pen-based user interfaces. It should be readily portable across platforms. It should support implementation of versions for languages other than English with minimal changes in programming. Because of variation in individual preferences, and also differing clinical and research needs and purposes, the ability to modify and customise the computer program is an important factor for individual users and research groups, as well as for further development of the SCAN system.

Visual display of information

In addition to the recording of ratings, the computer version must present data in a visually informative and clinically relevant way. The GUI (Graphic User Interface) program for the interview should show which items have already been rated, which have been scored positive, and which were absent or missed or could not be rated in spite of adequate inquiry. It should display diagnostic maps and allow manipulation of data to see the effects on the output of the algorithm.

The program should be able to present the course of symptoms in a graphical form, so that the clinician can perceive at a glance when a particular symptom or group of symptoms occurred. This would show longitudinal relationships that might otherwise be overlooked. The program should also be able to plot scores on groups of symptoms and represent different interviews, so that time changes in the SCAN profile of one individual, or of a group selected according to a particular characteristic, can easily be visualised.

Data management

A major advantage of computerisation is that it makes data handling easier. The program should be able to store information in a form that can readily be accessed by other programs for detailed statistical analysis, editing, amplification or modification. For security and confidentiality reasons the data should be encrypted and access allowed only by password. Different levels of security and access are necessary for administrative use. These and many other database functions can be implemented either by class libraries or rapid application development database systems. Class libraries provide a greater degree of flexibility and cross-platform portability but involve more complex lower-level design and programming. Database application development packages are available with many useful features, including varying degrees of cross-platform portability. Additional functions can be programmed in any of several compilers.

Networking and communications

The network of virtual communities of scientists and clinicians working together is increasing. This means that the program must allow easy networking and data transfer across local and wide area networks. Rapid developments in Web technology are making it feasible to connect databases to Web servers, allowing users easy interactive access to the underlying databases. These networking functions will support local as well as global data links, with the potential to make possible a worldwide real-time clinical psychiatric epidemiology. Research activities in general will be enhanced by such data systems.

Multimedia recording and playback

Standards for computer digital, audio and video recording exist and are rapidly becoming refined. Costs for necessary hardware are decreasing. The standards support the development of computer applications with these functions and the lowered costs make their widespread use practical. Development of the computerised SCAN should therefore include the incorporation of digital recording and playback functions. This will be valuable in research settings for reliability studies and for preserving non-verbal data in a convenient form, and in clinical settings for education, medical records and quality assurance.

Implementation

Programming methods

Given the issues outlined above, and particularly the central and critical nature of the database component of the computer application, efficient implementation of a reliable set of database functions is necessary. Many excellent rapid action development tools exist for this purpose. Although 16-bit operating systems (Windows 3.1) are still common, 32-bit systems are needed to fully exploit the possibilities for development. However there is already a substantial amount of control over the graphical interface, which allows the incorporation of digital multimedia functions.

Graphical interface

For ease of use a graphical user interface offers many advantages. Operation of the program can be more intuitive and natural compared to command line interfaces such as DOS. Another factor to be considered is the cost and existing availability of the hardware and operating system platform for a computerised version of SCAN. Microsoft Windows was chosen as the initial platform.

To make the computer SCAN familiar and easy to use, a visual desktop has been designed. However a computer desktop can provide more than a real one, since it can display various combinations of the SCAN Manual, Glossary, rating scales, previous episodes and maps of diagnostic algorithms and other subject data. The computerised SCAN also facilitates rapid navigation through its various components. Selection and movement to Part One or Part Two, sections, items and pages can be by keyboard entry, by mouse or by cursor keys. In future pen-based input will provide further efficiency.

The Glossary definitions are linked to the active item and thus automatically displayed. The Glossary window can be expanded to read long definitions more easily, or can be scrolled. Comments about the Glossary can be added and stored for subsequent reference. This feature is particularly useful for SCAN items with Glossary definitions that are incomplete or missing. This facilitates the SCAN tradition of openness to change, based on a wide consensus at regular intervals, meanwhile providing a standard that clinicians and researchers can use in order to promote comparisons, but from which they can also disagree and record their reasons.

Episode definition and item dating

Episode definition is an exercise in trade-offs in the printed SCAN, since multiple episodes create difficult formatting and space problems. The computer format, on the other hand, readily lends itself to the definition and documentation of multiple episodes. Dating of episodes and individual symptoms has also been somewhat problematic with the paper version. The computer version permits easy recording of the onset, termination and duration of key symptoms if the user so desires, as well as permitting the recording of the attribution of cause for individual symptoms. A pop-up calendar similarly provides ready reference to dates. For rating multiple episodes the rating window can be increased in size and can be configured by the user.

Item rating and notes

Rating scales are automatically linked to the current item. This avoids coding errors arising from the range of rating scales in SCAN. When a rating scale does not capture important aspects of the clinical situation, it is simple to record comments linked to the item and to retrieve these in context. This is an efficient equivalent to scribbles written on the printed SCAN or scoring forms. Such notes often contain ideas and thoughts that are forgotten minutes later by busy clinicians and researchers, but which (like suggestions for changes in the Glossary) can contribute to further evolution of the SCAN system. They will also be useful in a review of cases using the computer program. The presence of a comment is indicated by a flag on the rating box for the item (at the specified episode).

Longitudinal course

The ability of the SCAN computer application to create and use an unlimited number of episodes means that the Present State can be assessed repeatedly. Information on the Present State (usually the past month) is likely to be of better quality than the information obtained when trying to rate an episode many months or years ago.

Repeated Present State data over months or years can be analysed to provide improved understanding of the course of psychiatric conditions. One data-set of this kind contains paper observations on a group of 100 first onset psychosis patients in Madras who have been assessed monthly for over 10 years (Eaton et al., 1995; Thara and Eaton, 1996). Analysis of these data is yielding new insights into the course of schizophrenia, but is nevertheless limited by the sample size, the range of variables, the laborious nature of the data collection and massive work of data entry, checking and editing. The computerised SCAN will greatly help in this kind of research.

Configuration

The size of SCAN means that users may wish to use particular sections on their own. The computer application readily allows this. Users or research groups can configure the SCAN for a particular study, save the configuration and recall it when necessary. Items with insufficient Glossary definitions can be given extra specification in the Glossary window (see Item rating and notes above).

Manual data entry

Apart from the interview text and the Glossary, the program will have a separate module for entry of data from paper versions of the interview. Range checking for valid values is automatic. Standard double entry methods are supported. A timer function is built into the program which records time taken for the entry of each record. This will help users allocate time optimally for this process. The entry program permits the editing of earlier entries and also allows for double entries to check for errors in data entry. Earlier records can be opened and information for new episodes added.

Algorithm maps

A feature of the application is the operation of diagnostic algorithms for ICD-10 and DSM-IV. These operate on data entered manually or through the data entry interface. The user can select a data file and ask for a diagnostic output based on ICD-10 DCR or DSM-IV criteria. Options are provided to select the level of detail required from the analysis module. Results of the analysis can be stored in a file for review later. Users can also manipulate the status of a diagnostic algorithm at the SCAN item level without actually altering the already entered data. They can then observe the effects of the manipulations on the analysis. This also provides a more convenient method of checking diagnostic algorithms for errors.

Graphical maps of diagnostic tree structures are under development. Such maps would enhance the ability of SCAN users to recognise complex diagnostic relationships. It will be possible to map the relationships between ICD-10 and DSM-IV at the level of diagnosis, criterion or item.

Data files

The data file structure is designed so as to permit easy export of data into commonly used statistical packages, spreadsheets and other databases. This provides the user with the option of further data analysis without the burden of re-entering data. Global data warehouse considerations are also reflected in the data file structure.

Outputs

The computer application provides a variety of outputs to the user depending on individual needs. At the first level there is a textual output looking much like a clinical diagnosis, with a brief summary of the criteria met by the respondent according to ICD-10, DSM-III-R or DSM-IV, as selected by the user. The application will show a structural map for each diagnosis met. This includes the map of the diagnostic system chosen, the items in SCAN involved in that diagnosis, and the item ratings. In this way, the user can see the logic of the diagnostic algorithm. The user can also obtain online help in the form of the text of the diagnostic criteria, the SCAN item definitions and the level of the scores on each item. Navigation through the diagnostic system in order to display the maps for any diagnosis of choice, with full information as to why the respondent did or did not meet a particular diagnosis, will follow. The application will show the threshold requirements for individual SCAN items, at the level of criteria and at the level of the diagnosis. Thus the user can see, for example, which diagnoses would have been met had exclusion criteria been omitted.

User Feedback

Another useful note-taking function built into the SCAN computer application is a means for entering general comments on the program itself. This can include bugs, errors, and suggestions for improvement. The philosophy will be extended to Internet versions of SCAN and a community of SCAN Centers and users will thus become established.

Future development

This computer version of SCAN-2.1 follows the model of the printed SCAN but is able to solve many of its physical limitations. The virtual nature of the computer provides even more radical possibilities. Apart from the addition of audio and video recording and operation, the actual structure of SCAN can be unfolded and reorganised in many different ways, while preserving its core in the Glossary definitions and rating scales. For example, the separation of the interview manual from the Glossary has kept the manual from excessive unwieldiness, but produces inefficiency in referring to the Glossary. These two components are linked in the current computer CAPSE-2, but could be completely integrated in a future version. Conceptual developments and computer graphics can be combined to enhance the assessment of psychopathology. For example, the computer has the potential to bring the subject into greater participation in the assessment process, e.g. by displaying a life chart with significant events as an aid to temporal recall. A customised output for the respondent to look at and keep is another possibility providing a number of benefits.

It is envisaged that the suite of computer programs for SCAN-2.1 will serve as a foundation for computerisation of later versions as well as other assessment instruments. The international character of SCAN, the growth of the Internet and the design of the SCAN computer program have the potential to produce a global psychiatric database. Once this is achieved it may not be too unrealistic to envisage a worldwide virtual community of SCAN users connected on a network contributing to a shared database in real-time.

Implementation of computer algorithms will contribute to the understanding of algorithms used by clinicians. The process of developing computer algorithms requires continued decomposition and differentiation of the elements of clinical data and discovery of the cognitive processes used to analyse and synthesise the data. A clearer understanding of the thinking processes of clinicians would lead to more detailed and specific definition and measurement of psychopathology. This has implications for planned artificial intelligence and expert system additions to the computer SCAN.

The use of computers in psychiatry has been growing in both clinical and research areas, but with respect to diagnosis has been mostly a research activity. We think that the results of this research activity will have increasing application to clinical psychiatry, both in content and in method. The relevance of SCAN within a broader informatics context, including 'bottom-up' clinical data collected at the time of face-to-face contact with patients, patient self-report data (Brugha et al., 1996) computerised tests of brain function and 'top-down' information relevant to public health planning is manifest (Tien, 1997; Tien and Gallo, 1997; Wing, 1994).

References

American Psychiatric Association (1980) *Diagnostic and statistical manual of mental disorders*, third edition. Washington DC: APA.

American Psychiatric Association (1987) *Diagnostic and statistical manual of mental disorders*, third edition revised. Washington DC: APA.

American Psychiatric Association (1994) *Diagnostic and statistical manual of mental disorders*, fourth edition. Washington DC: APA.

Brugha, T. S., Kaul, A., Dignon, A., Teather, D. and Wills, K. M. (1996) PSE by microcomputer. Objectives and experience of preliminary steps. *International Journal of Methods in Psychiatric Research*, 6: 1–9.

Conrad M. (1993) Adaptability theory as a guide for interfacing computers and human society. *Systems Research*, 10: 3–23.

Dittman V. (1991) Modern psychiatric classification in research and clinical practice. *Schweitzer Archiv für Neurologie und Psychiatrie*, 142: 341–53.

Eaton W., Thara R., Federman E. et al. (1995) Remission and relapse in schizophrenia: The Madras longitudinal study. Submitted to *American Journal of Psychiatry*.

Feighner J., Robins E., Guze S. et al. (1972) Diagnostic criteria for use in psychiatric research. *Archives General Psychiatry*, 26: 57–63.

Jayaram G., Tien A., Sullivan P. et al. (1996) Salient elements of a successful short-stay service. *Journal of Psychiatric Service.* 47: 407–12.

Sartorius N., Kaelber C. T., Cooper J. E. et al. (1993) Progress toward achieving a common language in psychiatry: Results from the field trial of the clinical guidelines accompanying the W.H.O. classification of mental and behavioral disorders in ICD-10. *Archives of General Psychiatry* 50: 115–24.

Thara R. and Eaton W. (1996) Outcome of schizophrenia. The Madras longitudinal study. *Australia and New Zealand Journal of Psychiatry*, 30: 516–22.

Tien A. (1994) Computers, communication, and collaboration. In: G. Andrews, T. B. H. Dilling and M. Briscoe (eds.) *Computers in mental health*, vol. 1 Geneva: Longman Cartermill for WHO.

Tien A. (1997) Psychiatric epidemiology and information technology. *Psychiatric Annals*, 27: 268–72.

Tien A. and Gallo J. (1997) Clinical diagnosis. A marker for disease? *Journal of Mental and Nervous Disease*, 185: 739–47.

Üstün T. B. and Tien A. Y. (1995) Recent developments for diagnostic measures in psychiatry. *Epidemiologic Reviews*, 17, 210–20.

Wing J. (1994) A strategy for mental health informatics. In: G. Andrews, T. B. Üstün, H. Dilling and M. Briscoe (eds.) *Computers in mental health*. Geneva: Longman Cartermill for WHO.

World Health Organization (1992) *The ICD-10 classification of mental and behavioral disorders: clinical descriptions and diagnostic guidelines*. Geneva: WHO.

12 Clinical, educational and scientific uses

J. K. Wing, N. Sartorius and T. B. Üstün

Introduction: From PSE-9 to SCAN

The final chapter of the reference manual for PSE-9 was devoted to a discussion of its limitations and uses. The point made then remains true for SCAN/PSE-10. The advantages depend upon the disadvantages. It was pointed out that if SCAN was used within its limitations the advantages would be maximised. This apparent paradox is reconsidered in the context of changes made after more than 20 years of experience.

Limiting the limitations

Some of the limitations specified in the earlier manual have been rectified in SCAN. Cognitive dysfunction and decline are now covered sufficiently for use as part of a general psychiatric examination. Most other areas previously omitted from PSE-9, but now covered by the Diagnostic Criteria for Research of subchapters F1–F5 of ICD-10, are incorporated into SCAN. F6–F9 (personality disorders, learning disability, developmental disorders and problems arising in childhood and adolescence) raise different kinds of issues and separate instruments are required to address them. Provision is made for global ratings of key items in the Clinical History Schedule. These can be used as variables in the statistical analysis. The previous symptomatic history can now be recorded in substantial detail using CAPSE-2, and a much broader range of aetiological judgements, not available in the earlier system, is now supported in SCAN-2.1.

Other limitations were solved during the subsequent development of PSE-9 itself; e.g. the addition of an Index of Definition, supporting its use in population studies and in non-hospital settings as well as for in-patients. This will be adapted for use with SCAN, once trials have provided data according to which the final structure of symptom scores can be decided. Similarly, a set of symptom-type scores will need to be developed and tested on the basis of field trials.

The provision of detailed diagnostic criteria for ICD-10 and the DSM series solved another problem, since the criteria for ICD-8 were approximated from its prose descriptions and DSM-III was not then available. However, the caveat entered for CATEGO-4 remains valid for CAPSE-2, that the computerised diagnostic categories are not intended to be regarded as a full substitute for clinical diagnosis. Only a skilled clinician can assess the degree of a patient's co-operation, cognitive ability, facility with language and other factors affecting an interview and the ratings entered into a computer. If the ratings are trustworthy enough to be used as a basis for applying official (or other) diagnostic algorithms, that is the clinician's decision. If the system is used by someone without clinical skills, the categories derived from ratings cannot be regarded with the same confidence. The introduction of a short version of PSE-9, together with the Index of Definition, did demonstrate very useful results in population surveys, when used by non-clinical but skilled interviewers. Items requiring substantial clinical experience, such as obsessions, delusions, hallucinations etc., were omitted. It will be important to create and test an equivalent for PSE-10.

A limitation mentioned in 1974 that might still apply 'is that ratings of behaviour, affect and speech observed during examination are, on the whole, less reliable than those of subjectively described symptoms . . . This is probably due to the brief time sample available during examination, which means that severe examples are less likely to be observed.' The remedy then suggested, to use behaviour scales over a longer period of observation, remains apposite.

SCAN has not at present adopted a multiaxial classification, although the use of additional modules like IPDE for personality disorders, or the Disability Assessment Schedule for disability ratings, can cover some of the same functions. It will, however, be fairly simple to add an appropriate module once international agreement has been reached on the necessary structure.

A different kind of limitation can be viewed as a major advantage, in fact a necessity. SCAN has adopted a 'symptom oriented interview' that relies on 'cross-examination' of the respondent's experience in order to decide whether it fits a psychiatric symptom or sign defined in the Glossary. As a result, SCAN focuses on quantifiable phenomena to the extent that, by definition, it cannot itself provide a holistic understanding of the patient's personality, conflicts and life problems. The advantages of SCAN cannot be obtained without accepting the fact that it is not intended to cover the whole field of clinical work. One of its advantages is that it contributes an essential component without which no holistic understanding would be achievable.

Relationship of PSE-10.2 to earlier versions

A new limitation is that some sections of SCAN have changed so much since the field trials that further tests of reliability are needed. Areas affected include the somatoform, appetite, substance and cognitive disorders, and the attribution and context of causation. However, experience suggests that an acceptable level of reliability will be achieved across all these areas. This will still leave a major question as to the compatibility of the latest version with those that preceded it.

PSE-9

The most crucial difference between PSE-9 and all versions of PSE-10 is that the latter have been developed in relation to the two international (ICD and DSM) systems of diagnostic algorithms. Although many items are included that are not essential for either system, the need to keep to a reasonably sized instrument has meant that many PSE-9 items cannot be compared exactly with their PSE-10 'near-equivalents'. The extra rating point for many items (0–1–2 against 0–1–2–3) further exacerbates the problem, which conversion tables cannot easily solve.

The resulting lack of comparability is most serious when investigators wish to repeat (using PSE-10) studies of communities that have earlier been surveyed using PSE-9. Such studies have usually been designed in two stages, with the short form used during the first phase, and the full instrument administered to all those above the threshold for 'caseness' plus a sample of the rest. One way to make the comparison in a repeat survey would be to use PSE-9 (or its short form) for the first stage and PSE-10 appropriately interleaved with PSE-9 for the second. An experienced PSE interviewer would quickly learn to make the two sets of ratings. The resulting data would be useful not only for comparing estimates of morbidity over time but also for calibrating the differences between the instruments.

PSE-10.1

The differences between PSE-10.1/CAPSE-1, which has been used in some large-scale population studies, and PSE-10.2/CAPSE-2, are just as formidable though less obvious. The solution suggested for the equivalent PSE-9/10 problem might be too time-consuming to be practicable, but is worth trying.

PSE-10.2

Recent developmental work has centred on the need to provide software that would support the clinical administration and rating of PSE-10.2, together with the generation of ICD and DSM diagnoses. This preoccupation has meant that some elements of the broader 'SCAN' concept have not progressed to the same extent. These include the Symptom-type scoring system, the Item Group Checklist, the Index of Definition and the Clinical History Schedule, as well as the range of possibilities for making use of PSE-10.2 item profiles in conjunction with these higher-order elements.

These matters will form the next phase of development. Meanwhile it is important that this broader (bottom-up) context of SCAN should be kept in mind. The PSE has never been solely, or even primarily, an instrument for making a diagnosis.

Uses of SCAN: maximising the advantages

The aim of SCAN, set out in Chapter 3, is to provide comprehensive, accurate and technically specifiable means of describing and classifying clinical phenomena. Making comparisons is at the heart of all clinical, educational and scientific activities. The uses of SCAN, therefore, can be set out under these three headings.

Clinical

The first aim is to promote high-quality clinical observation. The instrument is designed to allow a comparison of the respondent's experiences and behaviour against the interviewer's Glossary-defined concepts, by a process of controlled clinical cross-examination. The resulting symptom profiles, scores and rule-based categories of disorder, can be compared with each other wherever in the world they are produced, and used for clinical audit, needs assessment and monitoring of progress of individual respondents. It is not necessary to agree with the concepts to be able to use their advantages fruitfully, within their limitations. A substantial clinical advantage is that many SCAN users comment that their style of interviewing, coverage and ability to recognise and describe psychopathology are improved even when they are not formally undertaking a SCAN interview.

Clinicians consider diagnosis as both a science and an art. Critical observation, and the generation and relevant testing of hypotheses, are aspects of the scientific method that should be applied routinely in clinical work. Making a single assessment using SCAN provides an opportunity to make comparisons with other patients known to the same clinician. Every interview and every prescription based upon it can be regarded as a clinical experiment. The educational and scientific uses are not therefore restricted to formal teaching of psychopathology and interview techniques or to formally designed research projects. Using the system makes it feasible to compare, and learn from, different clinical schools and to understand and apply the results of research more critically. The scientific aim is to accelerate the accumulation of knowledge by making all types of clinical experience, including education and research, more comparable, thus leading to more rapid agreement between groups on theoretical lines that could be useful for further advance.

A major clinical advantage is that the coverage of symptoms, signs and other relevant facts is not restricted to any one classificatory system. Criteria for ICD-10 subchapters F0 to F5, and the equivalents in DSM-IV are now almost completely covered down to 5-character level. But the ratings can be used to support any other diagnostic algorithm within this range if a list of system-specific items (e.g. different course criteria) is added. SCAN can easily be adapted to cover changes in diagnostic systems without altering any of its basic principles. Moreover, SCAN can be used in conjunction with a variety of other instruments and modules, covering, for example, conditions in subchapters F6–F9 of ICD-10.

A further advantage is the ability to make comparisons between diagnostic systems. This is most obvious in the case of ICD-10 and DSM-IV. When a PSE-10.2 protocol is fully completed, all the information for both systems is available for analysis. Applying the two sets of algorithms then allows the resulting diagnostic outputs to be compared and the reasons for any differences to be considered. The same could be true of any other set of diagnostic criteria that are created for particular purposes.

Educational

The second aim is educational and developmental; to improve clinical concepts by providing a common clinical language. The SCAN system contains the equivalent to a thesaurus of psychopathology, that can be linked to various sets of diagnostic criteria, at the moment covering ICD and DSM rubrics. It can therefore be used as a comprehensive aid to learning the basic elements of psychopathology and diagnostics. This makes it feasible to compare, and learn from, the usage of different schools. It is not necessary to agree with a common standard of reference in order to appreciate its value as a basis for communication and for comparison between different schools of clinical thought.

The further development of SCAN will benefit from such comparisons. New item-concepts will be added and old ones improved, preferably at carefully chosen intervals and with detailed updating instructions.

SCAN would also serve as an appropriate format for the standardised recording, storage and retrieval of diagnostic and classifying data internationally, as suggested in Chapter 11.

Scientific

All science is based on comparisons. The scientific value of SCAN lies in its potential to accelerate the accumulation of knowledge. Using standard technical procedures in research projects, such as the description of psychopathology, the measurement of change, standardisation of selection or the use of specifiable taxonomic systems, makes the results more precise and comparable, thus leading to more rapid agreement on useful theoretical lines for further investigation. This is true of all forms of research – biological, clinical, epidemiological, public health and psychosocial.

As the literature has amply demonstrated, SCAN/PSE-10 and its PSE precursors have been involved in virtually every aspect of clinically related research. There is a rich variety of first- and second-stage sample population studies, international comparisons, follow-up studies, controlled treatment trials, comparisons between instruments and investigations of biological, psychological and social causes. The list of references to 23 papers reporting studies using PSE-9 or SCAN, published in one professional journal during 1995 (see Appendix 2.1), is sufficient testimony to the usefulness of the procedures as aids to research. A full reference list is available from the Division of Mental Health, WHO, Geneva.

A less obvious contribution to learning and to science is the use of SCAN to study and improve techniques of measurement and classification. Its combination of 'bottom-up' phenomenology with 'top-down' categorisation, and the steady accumulation of a library of SCAN data-records at WHO, allows new approaches to classification to be tested.

Envoi: The future of SCAN

Since its origin in the late 1950s, the series of instruments that has culminated in the current Version 2.1 of SCAN, has evolved in a steady and consistent manner. Developed originally in the context of a tough and consistent school of psychiatry, tempered by the critical empirical approach natural to a research unit of the UK Medical Research Council, it developed into an international tool during the course of the US–UK Diagnostic Project and the International Pilot Study of Schizophrenia. There was a steady expansion of coverage. Experience with PSE-9 clearly demonstrated the applicability of the methods to epidemiological and public health surveys. It also indicated the need and demand for one or more handier versions to be used for specific purposes. SCAN contains many schedules that will in due course be made available as stand-alone or linked instruments as well as in the present format. CAPSE-2 has the potential to provide these.

Creating SCAN has brought together a network of people and institutions, which we hope will continue to develop in a creative way. The flexibility of the SCAN concept will allow its users to cope with whatever challenges are presented during the next century. For example, as specific laboratory techniques are developed to help diagnosis and classification, they can be incorporated into the SCAN system. New theories of causation, pathology and neurophysiology may well suggest combinations of clinical criteria very different from those in the current nosologies. But the symptoms and signs of mental disorder are unlikely to be much different from those now familiar to users of SCAN, and the bottom-up approach will remain the basis for clinical work.

Subject index